P9-DUP-310

WITHDRAWN
UTSA LIBRARIES

RENEWALS 458-4574

THE
QUALITY
IMPERATIVE

THE QUALITY IMPERATIVE

Measurement and Management of Quality in Healthcare

Editors

John R. Kimberly
University of Pennsylvania & INSEAD

Etienne Minvielle
CNRS, Paris

Imperial College Press

Published by

Imperial College Press
57 Shelton Street
Covent Garden
London WC2H 9HE

Distributed by

World Scientific Publishing Co. Pte. Ltd.
P O Box 128, Farrer Road, Singapore 912805
USA office: Suite 1B, 1060 Main Street, River Edge, NJ 07661
UK office: 57 Shelton Street, Covent Garden, London WC2H 9HE

British Library Cataloguing-in-Publication Data
A catalogue record for this book is available from the British Library.

THE QUALITY IMPERATIVE
Measurement and Management of Quality in Healthcare

Copyright © 2000 by Imperial College Press

All rights reserved. This book, or parts thereof, may not be reproduced in any form or by any means, electronic or mechanical, including photocopying, recording or any information storage and retrieval system now known or to be invented, without written permission from the Publisher.

For photocopying of material in this volume, please pay a copying fee through the Copyright Clearance Center, Inc., 222 Rosewood Drive, Danvers, MA 01923, USA. In this case permission to photocopy is not required from the publisher.

Library
University of Texas
at San Antonio

ISBN 1-86094-173-7

This book is printed on acid and chlorine free paper.

Printed in Singapore by FuIsland Offset Printing

Acknowledgments

This book is the result of a genuinely collaborative effort. In addition to the original contributions of the authors of the eight chapters that together form the core of the book, we would like to acknowledge the support of our institutions. The University of Pennsylvania and the Wharton School allowed John Kimberly to take the scholarly leave which made his work on the book possible. A heartfelt thanks, therefore to Tom Gerrity, then Wharton's Dean and to Janice Bellace, then Wharton's Deputy Dean, for their support. The Leonard Davis Institute of Health Economics and the French Institute for Culture and Technology at Penn provided support for the two conferences on quality in healthcare, one in Philadelphia in the summer of 1996, and one in Fontainebleau, France in the summer of 1997, which led to the writing of this book.

INSEAD, the European Institute of Business Administration, provided support in the form of a fellowship and visiting professorship to John Kimberly, financial and logistical support for the two quality conferences, and a grant from its R&D Fund to help with production of the book. A heartfelt thanks to Antonio Borges, INSEAD's Dean, and Hubert Gatignon, INSEAD's Associate Dean of Faculty, and to Landis Gabel and Luk van Wassenhove in their role as Associate Deans for R&D for their collective support of the development of *Healthcare2020* and healthcare management at the school.

The Ecole Nationale de la Santé Publique (ENSP) facilitated contact among the different research teams, while Karima Kaci and Valérie Landsmann of the Groupe Image at ENSP provided much of the logistical support required by the project. The Centre Nationale de la Recherche Scientifique (CNRS) provided a grant from its international cooperation program with the National Science Foundation to support the two quality conferences. Many other French organizations have contributed time and expertise, including the Assistance Publique-Hôpitaux de Paris and Institut National de la Santé Et de la Recherche Médicale (INSERM). A heartfelt thanks to Gérard de Pouvourville, then

v

scientific director of the Groupe Image-ENSP, who has been a source of continuous encouragement throughout the production of this book.

Our colleague Dr. Len Lerer, Research Fellow in *Healthcare2020*, INSEAD's initiative in healthcare management, in addition to contributing a chapter to the book also did yeoman's work in helping to edit and to format the entire manuscript.

To all of the above, we express our appreciation.

JRK and EM
Paris, June 1999

Contents

Chapter 1

Introduction: The Quality Imperative — Origins and Challenges

John R. Kimberly and Etienne Minvielle

Death in Surgery Reveals Troubled Practice and Lax Hospital. This headline on the front page of The Metro Section of the November 15, 1998 edition of The New York Times is followed by an article describing a routine surgical procedure which went very wrong and resulted in the death of a young woman. Subsequent investigation revealed a number of deficiencies in medical practice and in the hospital's policies which, together, created an environment in which "quality" of care might be compromised , in this case dramatically.

Les Bons Médecins. . .et Les Autres (The Good Doctors. . .and the Rest). Another headline, this time on the front page of the May 27, 1999 issue of Le Nouvel Observateur, a widely read French weekly newsmagazine. The accompanying article goes on to give the reader tips on how to choose "good" doctors and avoid the others and laments the fact that "En France aucune autorité n'a compétence à évaluer la qualité d'un médecin" (In France no formal body has the expertise to evaluate the quality of a physician).

These headlines and their accompanying articles—two from among literally hundreds that could have been cited—reveal much about the quality imperative in healthcare. Among the most salient features are:

Quality has become a very public issue (Lansky 1998). Whereas in the past, quality was controlled by the profession for the profession and was implicitly assumed to be non-problematic by the lay public, today this is no longer the case. Both of the publications cited above are

1

oriented to the public, and the fact that the articles discuss deficiencies brings the whole issue of quality to public attention in a singularly salient fashion.

Quality is becoming increasingly transparent, both within the profession of medicine and without (Bodenheimer 1999). Journals focusing on quality in healthcare have been established, professional associations dealing with quality are flourishing, media of all sorts feature stories about quality, "report cards" for physicians are being made public, and variability in quality of care from one hospital to the next is being measured and disseminated. Doctors are surrounded by quality initiatives and individuals, healthy and ill alike, are debating quality in the privacy of their living rooms, in public forums, and over the internet.

The management of quality in healthcare is becoming an increasingly global concern. Although widespread attention to quality management emerged initially in the United States, this concern diffused rapidly to other countries, as the headline from Le Nouvel Observateur suggests.

Quality in healthcare is complex and multi-faceted. The article from The New York Times suggests that quality is a function of an array of factors including the competence of medical professionals, the policies and procedures operative in the settings in which they practice, and the degree of vigilance that is exercised. The article from Le Nouvel Observateur, focused principally on doctors, notes that not all doctors are equally competent and suggests that individual patients should exercise caution when choosing a physician. The notion that individuals need to be proactive in managing their health status is relatively new, and adds another layer of complexity to the assessment of quality in healthcare.

Finally, the management of quality in healthcare is no longer the sole province of the medical profession. As both articles illustrate, each in a different way, the complexity of quality and the different interests that are at stake in its assessment and management require the involvement of multiple constituencies; payers, policy-makers, lay managers and patients—as well as physicians. No single party alone can be expected to "get it right"— whatever "getting it right" may mean.

Origins: The Heat Is On

As we have argued elsewhere (Kimberly 1997; Minvielle, de Pouvourville and Kimberly 1997), the worlds of medicine and healthcare are in a period of unprecedented transition in virtually every country around the globe, as essentially limitless wants confront the reality of limited resources. This confrontation raises the question of national priorities. Is there an upper bound to how much money countries are willing to spend on healthcare? How much is enough?

In country after country, governments have had to come to grips with questions of how to organize, finance and deliver healthcare in the context of competing priorities and concerns about increasing costs. Different answers are seen in different countries, to be sure, but no country is immune to the dilemmas that competing priorities pose. The heat, in other words, is on in the healthcare kitchen (Chassin and Galvin 1998), and enhancing efficiency, increasing professional accountability, and demonstrating value are the rallying cries of reform.

Enhancing Efficiency

The heat is on for enhancing efficiency. Given the multiple and competing pressures on governments in the resource allocation process, and given that these pressures are not likely to diminish, attention inevitably turns to how appropriately and judiciously existing resources are being used. Expenditures on healthcare in the developed countries range from just under 7% to over 14% of GDP (OECD 1998), and even though the differences across countries may be quite large, the absolute magnitude of the expenditures involved in all cases attracts attention and, in service of controlling costs, motivates questions about efficiency.

Responses have varied in their details from one country to the next, but are consistent in their emphasis on enhancing efficiency. Implementation of prospective payment in the United States, for example, changed the managerial incentives for hospitals dramatically, encouraging much closer scrutiny of the production process. Reforms currently underway in France in budgeting for health care will introduce similar incentives. The National Health Service in the UK has been experimenting with a variety of initiatives designed to encourage increased efficiency, as have many other countries in Western Europe. Predictably, these efforts have themselves spawned further questions, questions about the limits to efficiency. At what point do efforts to increase efficiency lead to problems with quality?

Increasing Professional Accountability

The heat is on to increase professional accountability. The profession of medicine has traditionally been central to healthcare systems around the globe. As the profession has matured, as its scientific knowledge base has become more specialized and differentiated, and as it has made spectacular inroads in curing the once incurable, most societies have accorded its high priests a degree of respect, prestige and professional license that is remarkable in its scope and pervasiveness. Physicians have historically had an extraordinary amount of control over the shape and surveillance of their profession. However, as the economics of healthcare have become increasingly problematic, questions have been raised about the way in which the profession itself and its work are organized, monitored and controlled. These questions have led to efforts to redefine, sometimes on the surface, but sometime more profoundly, the bases of organization, monitoring and control. Taken together, these efforts have created a new reality for the profession; it and its practitioners are being held to new and higher standards of accountability (Millenson 1997). Phrased differently, limits are being placed on the autonomy of physicians; they are increasingly being called upon to justify the decisions they make in the process of delivering care to their patients, decisions which have both medical and economic consequences (Newcomer 1998)

Demonstrating Value

The heat is on to demonstrate value. Purchasers of healthcare are becoming more sophisticated in their buying behavior and are beginning to insist upon "hard" evidence of value. No longer are they willing simply to write checks for services provided; they want to know what they are getting for their money and how it compares with what is available elsewhere. In the United States, initially the search for value translated into a search for lower prices. Or, more accurately, in an effort to keep costs in check, purchasers began to negotiate prices with providers, setting a wave of price competition in motion. Combined with the advent of prospective payment and managed care, these efforts led to a widespread public perception, reinforced by a number of highly publicized incidents, that the preoccupation with lowering costs was putting some people at risk of under- rather than over-treatment. To caricature the change only slightly, the concern shifted from the possibility that physicians were ordering too many tests and thus adding to costs unnecessarily to the possibility that physicians were ordering too few tests and thus jeopardizing the quality of care provided to patients.

In the midst of this maelstrom, purchasers began asking about value, that is, what benefits in terms of enhanced health status were being returned from dollars spent. They began, in other words, to demand that providers demonstrate value.

The Quality Imperative

At some level, quality has always been a concern in medicine in particular and in healthcare more generally. But the recent explosion of attention to quality is linked closely to the three rallying cries of reform described above. Efficiency cannot be enhanced until a baseline for efficiency is established. How many tests are too many? What is a reasonable standard for productivity? Increasing professional accountability is laudable, but for what should professionals be held accountable, how should the criteria be determined, and who should determine them? Demonstrable value is a reasonable criterion for purchase decisions, but how is it determined and by whom?

Responses to these three have converged in a way that has put the spotlight on quality. Quality has become the touchstone in debates about the organization, financing and delivery of healthcare. As such, it is invoked both by advocates of reform and guardians of the status quo. Reformers call for greater transparency in the name of improving quality, while their opponents caution against new initiatives in the name of preserving quality.

Behind and beyond the rhetoric, however, the quality imperative is evident in a multiplicity of efforts to bring light to heat, that is, to introduce systematic, data-based, consideration of quality into management in healthcare. These efforts fall into two general categories, efforts aimed at improving clinical quality of care provided (the **technical** dimension) and those aimed at improving the overall quality of the experience of providing and receiving care (the **process** dimension).

The Technical Dimension of Quality: Guidelines, Outcomes, and Evidence-Based Medicine

Medicine is a combination of art and science. The scientific portion of medicine, what we call the technical dimension, is that in which there is deep understanding of cause and effect relationships and where results are replicable on a continuing basis. Reliable judgements about quality can best be made where science is involved, that is, where research has demonstrated both an understanding of cause and effect and replicability of results. Under these circumstances, one can actually compare results, assess costs, and come to some reasonable and justifiable conclusion about value.

The recent flowering of interest in the development of clinical guidelines (Huttin 1997), in research on outcomes (Palmer 1997), and in evidence-based medicine (Drummond 1998) is testimony to the fact that medicine is coming of age and that informed judgements about quality are becoming and will increasingly become routine. This is not to say, however, that all of medicine is susceptible to the logic of scientific performance assessment, and one of the key issues for the future is determining which domains are most and least amenable to this logic. Indeed, one of the dangers in the current rush to quantify clinical quality is that the logic will be applied inappropriately in some instances. The scientific template and its associated tools and techniques should not be applied across the board. The costs of misapplication are potentially high, and may actually result in lowered rather than improved quality. Thus, although some very promising inroads have been made in assessing and improving quality in the technical dimension, much remains to be done and care must be used in judging where and how improvement efforts are applied.

TQM, CQI, and the Process Dimension of Quality

The second category of efforts to influence quality in health includes those aimed at improving the overall quality of the experience of giving and receiving care, what we call the process dimension (Berwick 1998). Among the initiatives that fall into this category are TQM, or "total quality management" and CQI, or "continuous quality improvement". These efforts, migrating into health care from the manufacturing sector of the economy, are broader in scope than the purely technical dimensions and touch on the way in which services are organized and delivered. The basic idea is that quality in all its complexity, ultimately resides in the concatenation of its constituent components. The managerial challenge, in this view, is, first, to recognize the many facets of quality, second, to work to improve as many of them as possible, but, third, to recognize their interdependence and the fact that they should not be managed piecemeal, but in concert.

The track record of many programmatic efforts in individual hospitals to introduce quality improvement is mixed at best (Arndt and Bigelow 1995; Carman, Shortell and Foster 1996). In our view, this mixed record in no way detracts from the underlying logic or potential benefits of the process-focused dimension of quality. Rather it speaks to the difficulty of implementing and institutionalizing a system-wide effort effectively and to the tendency of top management in health care establishments to search for "off-the-shelf", programmatic approaches. Although the desire to minimize the amount of managerial time and energy devoted to improving quality is certainly understandable given all of the other challenges faced, taking a superficial or cursory approach to implementation of quality improvement efforts has proved to be strikingly short-sighted. The emergence of quality as both a social good in itself and as a basis for determining value in the market for health care justifies (occasionally with hindsight) the investment in system-wide approaches.

Quality as an Important Social Good

In the context of the U.S., the importance of quality as a social good, a value which historically has been largely implicit, has become increasing explicit as criticisms of managed care have proliferated. More than any other single factor, the alleged excessive zeal of managed care companies in limiting care provided in service of controlling costs has propelled quality to the forefront of discussions of healthcare, health policy and the future (McLaughlin and Kaluzny 1997). There are intense debates, to be sure, about "how much" quality is enough at the societal level. And while it is undoubtedly true that some improvements in quality can be achieved without increasing costs, it is just as certain that at some point, improvements in quality can only be achieved with additional expenditures. Just how much any given society is willing or able to pay for given levels of quality is not obvious and the only certainty is that determining an answer will incite contention.

Quality as a Basis for Determining Value in the Market for Health Care

Implicit in the above discussion is the emerging belief that quality must play a more significant role in decision-making about healthcare, from the decisions that individuals make about where and from whom to seek care to decisions that payers make about the basis on which to purchase care. If there is social pressure to maintain some level of quality at the macro level, there is also economic pressure to seek value in healthcare transactions. This pressure comes from the recognition that cost alone is not a sufficient metric for determining value; quality must also be part of the value equation. Prudent and informed buyers in the market for health care, be they individuals or institutions, increasingly demand demonstration of value as an important component of their decision process. This, of course, means that providers must be in a position to show evidence of quality. It also means that evidence of quality can be used by providers as a basis for creating competitive advantage. Price competition alone is no longer an effective vehicle for doing so.

The search for value in healthcare is not restricted to "markets" in the narrow sense. It is emerging in many countries in Europe and elsewhere where national health insurance systems dominate. One consequence, of course, is that the determination of quality has become a preoccupation, and efforts to develop reasonable measures and the associated information infrastructures to support it have become big business.

The Challenge of Managing Quality

These factors together—the desire to enhance efficiency, to introduce new and higher standards of professional accountability and to demonstrate value—

have led to a genuine explosion of interest in both the technical and the process dimensions of quality (Chassin and Galvin 1998; Thomson, 1998). One result of the emergence of the quality imperative is an accumulating body of evidence about the challenges that go along with managing quality systematically and consistently. We visit this evidence in more detail in the final chapter, but for present purposes, we would like to highlight the following implications:

The management of quality must be sensitive to the **special character of healthcare**. Once cannot simply import and replicate models from industry.

The management of quality should be approached **systemically**, rather than in piecemeal fashion.

The management of quality must involve **all** parties—physicians, nurses, managers, support staff and patients.

The management of quality must be a **strategic priority** for the institution.

The management of quality must include both the **technical** and **process** dimensions.

The Plan of the Book

The various chapters in this book all speak directly to the quality imperative and to the challenge of measuring and managing quality in healthcare in an era of rapid change and heightened pressures for performance. The book is divided into three sections, **Perspectives**, **Practices**, and **Potential**.

Part I, **Perspectives**, consists of two chapters that together provide an overview of the terrain and point out specific areas of particular emphasis. Chapter 2, by Gérard de Pouvourville, places information at the heart of quality improvement efforts. In describing the emergence of concern with quality in the U.S. and France, he shows how dependent any systematic approach to the problem is on the availability of appropriate information. Chapter 3, by Dominique

Tonneau, approaches quality from the perspective of its organizational and managerial implications. Based on extensive research and consulting experience in hospitals, he emphasizes that physicians have always been concerned with quality—what is new is the organizational dimension.

Part II, **Practices**, consists of four chapters, each of which describes and analyzes actual efforts to manage quality in France and in the U.S. Chapter 4, by Martin Charns and his colleagues, reviews the results of an extensive study of "programming" and "feedback" approaches to coordination in surgical services in the Veterans Administration system in the United States and their impact on patient care outcomes. They find that the two approaches are additive, that is, use of both simultaneously improves patient outcomes in the surgical services they studied. Chapter 5, by Robin Gillies and her colleagues presents the results of a study of Continuous Quality Improvement efforts in coronary artery bypass graft surgery and total hip replacement in 16 hospitals in the United States. The conclusions are sobering; the investigators found implementation of CQI to be fraught with challenges, challenges that they describe in some detail. Their chapter raises serious questions about just how much real change can be expected from investment in CQI.

In Chapter 6, Isabelle Durand-Zaleski and Pierre Durieux describe the current context of quality improvement efforts in France and discuss experiences with the development of what they call "Evaluation Units". Although the details are different, one cannot but be struck by the many similarities between the challenges they describe and those chronicled in the previous chapter by Gillies and her colleagues. Finally, in Chapter 7, David Shulkin and Maulik Joshi take us inside the University of Pennsylvania Health System for a look at how a large, complex provider has approached the measurement and management of quality. Given the difficulties in the implementation of quality improvement efforts rehearsed in the previous two chapters, this chapter provides an interesting contrast. Despite the challenges, the UPHS has successfully implemented their approach to quality management, and in so doing, has created a model from which others might learn.

Part III, **Potential**, consists of three chapters, each looking at the measurement and management of quality in healthcare prospectively. Chapter 8, by Jon Chilingerian, proposes that efforts to measure quality should focus on outliers rather than central tendencies. This change, he argues, should move institutions more surely in the direction of best practice and would thus have the greatest impact on quality. Chapter 9, by Len Lerer, is critical of current efforts to deal with quality and proposes instead what he calls a "putative framework", one which emphasizes the importance of context in influencing outcomes. This newer framework, he contends, will force managers to look beyond purely mechanical approaches and to focus instead on sustainable improvement. In the concluding chapter, Etienne Minvielle and John Kimberly review and synthesize the previous chapters and sketch out an agenda for quality management in the future.

Quality Management is Here to Stay

David Eddy (1998) has argued that "performance measurement is here to stay" in healthcare. We would agree with Eddy's contention, and would argue further that "quality management is here to stay". The stakes, both social and economic, are simply too high for it to be otherwise. The search for value by purchasers will continue, and as it does, more refined ways to measure and manage quality will be developed. The chapters in this book suggest both what has been accomplished thus far and what remains to be done. The quality imperative is real, and to respond intelligently to the imperative is one of the most pressing challenges facing the health sector.

References

Arndt, M., and B. Bigelow. 1995. The Implementation of Total Quality Management in Hospitals: How Good is the Fit? *Health Care Management Review* 20(4):7-14.

Berwick, D. 1998. Crossing the Boundary: Changing Mental Models in the Service of Improvement. *International Journal for Quality in Health Care* 10(2):435-41.

Bodenheimer, T. 1999. The American Health Care System—The Movement for Improved Quality in Health Care. *New England Journal of Medicine* 340:488-92.

Carman, J.M., S.M. Shortell, and R.W. Foster. 1996. Keys for the Successful Implementation of Total Quality Management in Hospitals. *Health Care Management Review* 21:48-60.

Chassin, M.R., and R.W. Galvin. 1998. The Urgent Need to Improve Health Care Quality. *Journal of the American Medical Association* 280:1000-5.

Drummond, M. 1998. Evidence-based Medicine and Cost-Effectiveness: Uneasy Bedfellows. *American College of Physicians Journal Club* 3:133-4.

Eddy, D.M. 1998. Performance Measurement: Problems and Solutions. *Health Affairs* 17(4):7-25.

Huttin, C. 1997. The Use of Clinical Guidelines to Improve Medical Practice: Main Issues in the United States. *International Journal for Quality in Health Care* 9 (3):207-14.

Kimberly, J. R. 1997. Assessing Quality in Health Care: Issues in Measurement and Management. *International Journal for Quality in Health Care* 9(3):161-2.

Lansky, D. 1998. Measuring What Matters to the Public. *Health Affairs* 17(4):40-41.

McLaughlin, C .P., and A. D. Kaluzny. 1997. Total Quality Management Issues in Managed Care. *Journal of Health Care Finance* 24 (1):10-16.

Millenson, M. L. 1997. *Demanding Medical Excellence.* Chicago: University of Chicago Press.

Minvielle, E., G. de Pouvourville, and J. R. Kimberly. 1997. Introduction: Les Demarches Qualite a l'Hopital. *Gestions Hospitalières* 369:611-12.

Newcomer, D. 1998. Physician Measure Thyself. *Health Affairs.* 17 (4):32-5.

OECD. 1998. *OECD Health Data 1998.* Paris: Organization for Economic Cooperation and Development.

Palmer, R. H. 1997. Using Clinical Performance Measures to Drive Quality Improvement. *Total Quality Management.* 8 (5):305-11.

Thomson, R. G. 1998. Quality to the Fore in Health Policy — At Last. *British Medical Journal.* 17:95-6.

Part I.   Perspectives

Chapter 2

Information Systems and Quality in Health Care

Gérard de Pouvourville

Over the past twenty years, health services have been under growing external pressure to become more accountable, initially to payers, but increasingly to all levels of government, law courts and patients. Although cost-containment pressures may have precipitated the accountability debate, the scope of accountability has widened to include quality. The quality argument is used by health professionals, who resist resource constraints by arguing that these would reduce the quality of patient care. Providers use quality as a marketing tool in an increasingly competitive environment. The intensity and modalities of the pressure to be accountable have been influenced by factors such as different national institutional settings, trust placed in providers, and the degree of concern about health expenditures and quality of care. In Europe, competition between health insurance companies and providers plays a lesser role than in the United States. European governments and administrative bodies, are the primary participants in the quality debate and regulation is the main tool to ensure quality of care (de Pouvourville 1997).

National characteristics are important as they, more or less, define the constraints and opportunities for quality of care initiatives. However, there is also a strong belief that health care technology (the broad combination of competencies, human and technical resources used in the delivery of health services) differs little between most developed countries. This contention is strengthened by the "globalization" of health and life sciences research, as well as the market for drugs and equipment. Moreover, all developed countries are participants in the "information revolution". Finally, in industrialized countries, there exists a strong belief that the rationalization of work processes is a valuable end to be attained. Despite major differences in the way that

15

health care is organized, financed and managed at a country level, there is an international "market for ideas" that plays an important role in the diffusion of managerial innovation (Kimberly and de Pouvourville 1993). There is no doubt that such a market exists for quality of care and related information management tools. The major players are health care decision makers, either regulators, managers or providers looking for solutions to their problems, consulting firms trying to expand their market, computer companies selling integrated services, and academics seeking research opportunities.

How does one become a clever buyer in such a market, when the product is complex, incorporating information and communication technologies, analytical tools and managerial models? I shall try to answer this question, by sketching an analytical framework of information systems dedicated to the assessment of quality in health care. This framework focuses on organizational, "political" and human resource issues, as opposed to purely an assessment of information technology.

What is Quality of Care?

The Office of Technology Assessment (1993) defined the quality of a provider's care as "the degree to which the process of care increases the probability of desired patient outcome and reduces the probability of undesired outcomes, given the state of medical knowledge". Although this definition may seem quite general and difficult to operationalize, a detailed analysis yields some important insights.

The definition of quality indicates that when comparing two providers taking care of exactly the same patient population, one is providing a better quality of care if his percentage of patients with positive outcomes is higher than that of the other. Similarly, a better quality provider has a lower percentage of patients with negative outcomes. Most importantly, this definition of quality focuses on outcomes; that is health status after care has been delivered. This definition appears to be relevant to the current situation, since it emphasizes the need to measure the outcome of care. This has obvious consequences for information systems, as it requires that priority be given to the follow-up of patients and their health status over time.

A second aspect of this definition relates to the validity of comparisons. One can compare one provider with another, only if both have the same types of patients. This highlights the importance of defining case-mix by identifying those patient characteristics that have an impact on outcome. This also has important implications for information systems, since the correct adjustment of case-mix and severity requires detailed clinical data, which increases the cost of information.

Thirdly, the term *desired* (and undesired) raises the question of who sets the level of desirability required. Although quality of care was traditionally a professional issue, this situation has changed dramatically. Payers pressure providers to reduce costs while improving outcomes. Payers have also attempted to reframe the traditional equation that states that increasing cost is an inescapable result of improved quality. The opinions of patients should also be elicited when considering the desired level of quality of care. Patients and physicians do not share the same perception of risk and often differ on what level of intervention constitutes the most appropriate care. Lebeer (1997) has shown how patients refusing painful cancer therapy are considered as "psychologically deviant" by caregivers. Such patients often receive psychiatric care, when simply expressing a personal value judgement on pain versus the hypothetical benefits of therapy.

Fourthly, the definition does not explain the avenues available to improve quality. As previously mentioned, it focuses mainly on outcomes. We need to clarify the inherent differences between quality primarily as an outcome issue (outcome quality), and quality as a process issue (process quality). The measurement of outcome, that is the improvement in health status after an intervention, may be difficult and costly even when restricting the analysis to clinical data. As desirable outcomes include a rapid return to functional status and the long-term absence of complications, measurement requires longitudinal follow-up of patients. To deal with this, physicians rely on controlled and uncontrolled trials that allow them to make explicit assumptions about the relationship between process and outcome quality. These assumptions have obvious economic advantages in terms of information systems, because, as careful process control is vital in health care delivery, there is no need to expend resources to assess outcomes. Health care delivery is a complex activity, as the "product" combines medical treatment, interpersonal relationships and aspects of the service industry. As it is difficult to establish a direct relationship between process quality and outcomes, intermediate measures of outcome are used. Intermediate outcomes must not be mistaken with the final outcome, which is a sustained improvement in health status. The concept of quality in health care has two facets. On the one hand, quality is an outcome issue, and as such must include some form of value judgment on the desirability of specific outcomes, not only by providers, but also by society as a whole. On the other hand, because outcome measurement is difficult, quality of care is regarded as the result of the process of care. Although it may be acceptable to use process quality as a proxy for outcome quality, this link does not always exist and it is important to maintain the analytical distinction between the two. From an economic standpoint, quality of care as an attribute of outcome relates to allocative efficiency, since it requires value judgments on outcomes.

Quality of care as an attribute of process is related to technical efficiency. Given the value of a treatment, how can it be delivered with the best combination of resources? In terms of information systems, such a concept of quality has specific implications. Firstly, notwithstanding difficulties with follow-up, all information collection efforts should be devoted towards outcomes. Secondly, outcomes should include some measure of value that is important to patients. Thirdly, it is acceptable to substitute process for outcome when enough evidence exists to show a direct positive relationship between the two, but it should be kept in mind that this is not an optimal solution. Fourthly, we require good controls for case-mix to facilitate comparisons between providers. Finally, quality of process must be measured on all dimensions of service including clinical care, patient satisfaction, administration and logistical issues.

The Nature of Information Systems

An information system can be broadly defined as the set of cognitive resources used by actors in an organization to assess a situation, choose an action, implement it, evaluate it and account for it. Because of the wide range of tasks and controls, different parts of an organization can have different information systems. Thus, the general term "information system" should not lead us to believe that consistent applications are possible within organizations.

By considering information as a cognitive resource, we are adopting an analytical standpoint that separates the value of the information from the context of the interaction between actors. With this caveat in mind, information systems are usually composed of infrastructure to record and transmit information, languages and cognitive routines of analysis. The physical infrastructure can be a mix of computers, paper files, communication systems, and human brains, the collective memory of employees being a major component of information systems in organizations. Vendors usually emphasize the computer hardware and software systems, but the value-adding potential of technological innovation is highly dependent on the implementation process.

Languages can be quite diverse, informal and sometimes based on visual or auditory signals. The transmission of information on a large scale usually requires the standardization of languages, in general through coding schemes. Cognitive routines of analysis are a major component of an information system. and the adoption of information technology allows us to deal with decision making in an innovative fashion. Organizations, anticipating the changes that come with new information technology, may accept or resist innovation. A critical factor supporting adoption of information systems is the opportunity for members of an organization to develop their own new and improved work-routines.

Thus, information systems are at the crossroad of three major technologies, which interact with one another: the technology of information processing, the technology of health care and outcomes measurement, and the technology of operations management and workflow control.

Information Systems in Health Care

What types of information systems can be observed in the health care delivery systems of developed countries? Economic activity requires a minimum level of infrastructure to define the transactions between providers and purchasers and to permit contracting and payment. This infrastructure is a mix of formal, explicit requirements and more implicit conventions, built up, over time, as common and frequently tacit knowledge. Traditionally, medical professionals have been responsible for defining the frequency, duration and context of transactions in health care delivery. The epidemiology and implications of illness and the complexity of health care have resulted in public authorities, insurers and doctors playing a major role as surrogates for consumers. In this context, information systems have developed mainly to assist in the interaction among these parties and have been based on nomenclatures and service classifications, such as medical procedure lists. As the United States, more than most developed countries has a system of competition between insurers and providers and a strong tradition of health related litigation, health information systems have always had to be extremely detailed. For example, the recording of diagnosis data on a routine basis for each hospital stay has been compulsory in the United States for over thirty years, while in several European countries; this is not yet the case. In France, it is only since 1996 that the coding of procedures, for primary care physician claims, was made compulsory, although this has not yet been implemented. It not possible to judge the impact of innovation on the health care consumer—the patient. One can only observe that other national systems facing resource constraints, are adopting information systems resembling those found in the United States, without necessarily moving towards competition among private insurers and the private provision of services.

Public health information systems have a specific function. They are based on the idea that it is the responsibility of public authorities to ensure that determinants of health, such as water, sanitation and waste removal, both prevent epidemics and improve health. Public health authorities also have to evaluate the organization of health care itself, against benchmarks of equity and access to good quality care. Administrative data, available to public health physicians can provide insights into the variability of medical practice and disparities in the health system. In general, such data are provided by surveys designed to address a specific public health issue, but may also be available from routine records. There is considerable debate about whether specific information systems for health services research, as opposed to the use of routinely available administrative data, are necessary. In general, large routine databases do not include detailed clinical information and data permitting assessment from the patient's perspective (McGlynn 1997). Indeed, there seems to be a gap between the sophisticated research on quality measurement and the evolution of health care organization information systems. Thus, administrative databases can be used to detect problems, but may not be sufficient to permit in-depth investigation. Large databases often have a greater proportion of inaccurate records and the data may not be categorized in a way that allows easy analysis of a quality problem. Large databases, however, provide the framework within which focused surveys can be conducted.

In response to increased external pressure for accountability, providers have developed internal information systems that mirror the requirements of public regulators and payers. These systems directly determine the internal incentives and modalities of control within provider organizations, such as hospitals. Although these systems permit the identification of major areas of inefficiency, they cannot provide service delivery solutions. Providers, forced to demonstrate gains in efficiency, are seeking solutions used in other industries. The need for alternative organizational structures and management methods has boosted the market for information systems oriented towards initially, utilization review and quality assurance, and more recently, total quality management.

In all developed countries, increased coordination or integration of care has been seen as the key to cost-containment. France, for example, has used financial incentives to encourage networking between hospitals, specialists and primary care physicians in areas such as AIDS, diabetes management and perinatal care. Within these networks, information systems are assumed to facilitate communication between providers in order to coordinate and rationalize care.

Finally, the progress of communication technology has resulted in large, ambitious health informatics projects using the internet and smart cards. Starr (1997) reported on the fate of community health management information systems in the USA, arguing that there was not enough value added for competitive providers to network and centralize all health care data for a given area. The internet offers more flexibility and proprietary systems may facilitate competitive advantage previously associated with exclusive data access. In France, the government has recently launched a National Network for Health and Social Services, the RSS, dedicated exclusively to health care professionals (de Pouvourville, Andral and Lombrail 1999). Access to the RSS is controlled by a smart card and the network allows for the electronic processing of claims. It is expected that the network, operated by a private company under public contract, will permit collection of data on the use of health services and improve quality of care through better communication among health care providers. The RSS was created under the assumption of a natural monopoly based on the security of transactions with the smart cards, but it now appears that private networks can offer the same level of security with other technologies.

Information Systems and Economic Incentives in Health Care

Information systems were developed in part as a provider response to increasing pressure from payers, initially for cost containment and more recently for quality. In the case of professional behavior, we can distinguish between two different philosophies of external control. The first relies on case-by-case analysis of medical practice, to pinpoint and penalize "inappropriate" practices. One could describe this model of control as external and bureaucratic, as it relies on the idea that medical practice can be standardized. The second philosophy is based on the principle that medical practice can only be standardized to a certain limited extent, and that professionals should have some decision making discretion, if only to take patients' preferences into account. This philosophy also considers that professionals should be accountable for their practices, in terms of cost and quality. Under such a model, external control is through global economic incentives such as capitation and internal control is exercised through accreditation, defined as self-policing within professional organizations.

The mechanism of exclusively external control forces health care providers to provide payers with extensive information on each patient interaction, including medical data. Indeed, payment systems based on fee-for-service result in complex information systems, since they require the production of a claim for every patient contact. When control is exerted through overall expenditure ceilings, specific claims data may not be required. Although the payer may have some access to the provider's internal information system, specific data on each patient interaction may not be available. Health services researchers in the USA are concerned that capitation may result in the loss of case-specific discharge data, a valuable tool for assessing quality of care.

What determines the level and extent of control in a health system? One assumption is that this may be partly dependent on macroeconomic factors that shape a national health system, and particularly, on the extent to which payers can control expenditures (Develay, Naiditch and de Pouvourville 1996). For example, in the USA, there is no overall macroeconomic mechanism to control the level of health sector expenditure. The system is economically decentralized and it is left to multiple payers to limit provider charges, control costs and gain competitive advantage. Under these conditions, the development of information systems is a necessary condition to normalize transactions and monitor professional practices. On the other hand, in the United Kingdom, the overall level of expenditure is nationally controlled, since health services are financed through taxes. Expenditure controls are exerted through capitation for primary care, and hospital budgets. Health care reform in the United Kingdom was primarily driven not by cost containment concerns, but rather by the lack of provider responsiveness to patients needs and problems with access to specialized, hospital based care. The reforms introduced at the beginning of the 1990's aimed to improve access to specialist care, by allowing primary care physicians to purchase care, and introduced competition among hospitals, based on quality of service. For primary care physicians, this arrangement meant accountability for expenditures made on behalf of their patients, but it did not result in the introduction of quality monitoring or utilization review. In principle, the contracts with hospitals should have resulted in a demand for information to monitor hospital physician practices. What happened instead was that hospitals were obliged to develop billing systems and communicate discharge abstracts to primary care physicians, although this information was not used to monitor practices. Waiting times for investigations and surgery have become important quality issues, but the assessment of the quality of medical care, in the United Kingdom, remains an implicit and informal transaction between physicians.

Information Systems and the Management of Quality

A dual philosophy of control can also be observed in the evolution of provider information systems and their utilization to promote quality of care. The role of information systems ranges from being a method to assess quality retrospectively to a system for integrating quality into the production process.

Initially, hospitals, mainly in the United States, responded to external pressures through the implementation of Utilization Review (UR), and later Quality Assurance (QA) programs. UR generally refers to the economics of the process, that is the quantity of resources used. In order to avoid a situation where the control of resources takes precedence over access and the appropriateness of care, resource allocation needs to be linked to certain basic requirements for medical care. The role of QA is to define such requirements and to design and implement methods to assess whether an institution is meeting these requirements. We can see that UR and QA are closely linked and that

QA should theoretically and ethically dictate the nature of UR procedures. Information requirements for QA and UR programs are determined by choices made on the following dimensions:

Levels of data and tools required: Schumacher (1989) identifies four levels of data and measurement tools in a hospital information system. Each level corresponds to a category of stakeholder and type of decision. The first level is strategic: it is related to the overall policy of the institution. Examples of data and tools needed are product lines and market penetration, and proxies for quality such as crude mortality rates or patient satisfaction indices. The second level is operational: this relates to the appropriateness of resource allocation amongst the various product lines, as may be measured by patient classification systems. At this level, severity adjusted mortality rates, analysis of case mix and departmental budgeting based on costs per case, are appropriate data. The third level is the routine management of the processes in care units. Relevant data are patient and clinical data from the medical record, and cost data from the cost accounting system. Finally, the fourth level corresponds to the "fine-tuned" assessment of care or clinical research.

Scope of programs: UR and QA programs may encompass a variety of aspects of institutional performance. For example, the credentialing policy of a hospital may be part of a QA program. Such programs should include the working relationship of a hospital with its environment, such as ambulatory care and links with other institutions.

Definition of standards: UR and QA methods need reference standards to benchmark practice patterns. Such standards may be norms set according to the objectives of a specific institution (for example, length of stay standards set by payers, or admission criteria for certain units). The standards may also be set through professional peer review and can be validated through empirical studies (randomized controlled trials, meta-analysis, and experimental databases).

Data focus: Donabedian (1989) distinguishes three levels of focus in the analysis of the quality of care: structure, process and outcomes. He notes that it is difficult to infer anything about quality of care from data on structures alone, and that processes may be defined implicitly (case review by experts) or by using explicit criteria, which is more costly, but more reliable. The measurement of outcomes is difficult, because outcome is a multi-dimensional concept and ideally, "outcome measures should be tied to process measures that point directly to specific steps that can be taken to improve care"(Chassin, Kosecoff and Dubois 1987)

Types of data analysis: There are two main types of analysis: a case-by-case analysis (for example, the analysis of a small random sample of medical records) or population based analysis (for example, the analysis of all surgical cases).

Timing of data collection: Data can be collected on a routine, permanent basis, on a routine, periodic basis, or on an ad-hoc basis in response to identified problems.

Timing of the use of data: Data can be analyzed and used immediately to monitor the care process, or on a retrospective basis, to evaluate performance and identify problems.

Generally, UR and QA programs constitute a mixture of the aforementioned dimensions, according to the objectives of the programs and the nature of the change process. The information methodologies used by UR and QA programs fall into four main categories:

The first category constitutes crude, uni-dimensional indicators, loosely related to each other and analyzed retrospectively to identify potential problems. Examples are length of stay data, crude mortality rates, premature discharge rates, surgical complications rates and hospital-acquired infection rates. Although such indicators assist in identifying issues requiring urgent attention, they do not provide much guidance on appropriate remedial action.

The second category refers to screening methods, which also rely on a series of crude indicators, but focus on the immediate identification of problems that can further be analyzed through prospective and retrospective studies. Screening usually concentrates on a narrow sequence of events in the process of care. Quality assurance programs in American hospitals are based on screening methodology and the variables are often locally defined, or are developed to respond to particular institutional requirements. Information required is generally available from various sources (specific spreadsheets, nurses' logbooks or care plans, and medical records), and the interpretation of the data relies heavily on the available documentation and on the experience of the person (usually a nurse) in charge of the UR or QA program.

A third category is the existing patient classification schemes (PCSs). As compared to simple indicators or screening methods, PCSs have the advantage of being able to cope with the variability of case mix, and thereby distinguish between the burden of illness (in particular, the severity of illness) and patterns of medical practice. They are thus a powerful tool to enhance the results yielded by simple indicators and screening, since they allow a clinically meaningful presentation of the data and their interpretation in terms of utilization or quality. Finally, as aggregate measures, PCSs permit the analysis of trends over time, comparisons between providers, and small area variation analysis of hospital resources and procedures (Kazandjian et al. 1989; Winickoff et al. 1984). PCSs may be solely process oriented (DRG, PMC), process and outcome oriented,(CSI, Medisgrp, APACHE), or disease oriented (ICD, Disease Staging).

Detailed, specific clinical data are the last category. They are required for risk-adjustment and whenever an in-depth analysis of practice is undertaken. Information is usually available on the medical records of patients, but if such records are not computerized, routine use of such data to assess quality is quite costly.

External agencies remain concerned with the identification of cost outliers, inappropriate admissions and procedures for which they may be able to deny payment. This interest in individual cases has led to the development of auditing methods to sample medical records. Since it is difficult for hospitals to design a computerized information system able to respond to a wide range of sampling requirements, analysis often requires the manual extraction of data which are discarded after use. Consequently, there is no incentive to develop systems allowing for long-term performance trend analysis, based on hospital utilization and outcomes data (Roper 1989). Moreover, the various standards developed by the different agencies lack specificity in terms of the assessment of appropriateness of care, and may thus be contradictory. The emphasis on UR has also underscored access issues and the maldistribution of procedures and care, all of which are critical dimensions of quality. Another impact of UR in the United States has been growing public suspicion of physician skills and practices resulting in increasingly difficult working conditions in hospitals and more malpractice litigation.

In reaction to this coercive process, new concepts and implementation paradigms have emerged under the label of "continuous quality improvement" or "total quality management". The emphasis is now on systems versus individuals and the management of quality is regarded as part of the daily care process. The emphasis is put on the overall organization of care and on all patients, not only the outliers. This approach stresses prevention as opposed to the retrospective detection of faults. Attaining continuous process quality requires that overall performance standards be set and trends simultaneously monitored to detect variations from the norm. Information technology is a necessary tool to achieve the goal of continually monitoring the process of care and assessing its quality.

Fortunately, technological progress has continued in many dimensions. The speed, capacity and availability of computers have increased substantially and lower unit prices make widespread computerization possible in most health care organizations. Networking technology has also multiplied the potential for interaction between different actors, and electronic technologies for the control of workflow, such as bar-coding, have emerged. The capacity to track products or people as they move through a facility reduces waiting times, improves coordination and permits rapid reaction to variable conditions. Changes in management philosophy and technology have resulted in the demand for information systems that are more oriented towards real-time monitoring of the workflow around the patient.

Concluding Comments

Health care systems in developed countries have entered a new era. The traditionally wide scope of responsibility accorded to professionals is progressively being replaced by a more equitable relationship among providers, payers, patients and public authorities. Measurement of the value-added by health care services, inconceivable until recently, is now considered not only feasible, but also imperative. The complexity of medical care is no longer an obstacle to its objective assessment, in part because professionals themselves have led the way towards an evidence-based rationalization of medical practice. Information technology has played a major role in this transformation, as it has opened large databases to scientific scrutiny.

The transformation of health care has not been linear, nor has it been homogeneous within national systems or between different countries. There is still strong opposition to broadening the range of stakeholders in health sector decision making, as this threatens the autonomy of health care workers. Data analysis methods and performance indicators still require further development and databases are costly to maintain. The transformation of the health sector has caused us to reconsider the efficiency of care and question the management of provider organizations. It was initially assumed that as practices could be standardized, a bureaucratic approach to professional control was appropriate. Industry, however, had realized that formal rules and control were not the solution in a rapidly changing, competitive environment. Moreover, if relevant quality measures were to be available, cooperation with professionals was a necessary condition for success (Hannan et al. 1994). Thus, the story of information systems in health care mirrors the organizational model of each period, the existing technologies, and the major methodological progresses in the development of quality measures.

Clearly, the exigencies of the health sector are different from those of the industrial sector and industrial quality approaches need to be adapted for use in health care. What is required is the recognition of the centrality of professionalism and a radical change in the interaction between physicians and other health care professionals with the ultimate objective of creating flexible organizations, oriented towards the continuous management of quality. Well-designed information systems, reflecting the best organizational models, existing technologies and innovations in health services research, are essential in the transition towards quality.

References

Chassin, M., J. Kosecoff, and R. Dubois. 1987. *Value-managed health care processing project, Volume 2*. Chicago:Midwest Business Group on Health.

Develay, A., M. Naiditch, and G. de Pouvourville. 1996. Information médicale et régulation de la médecine générale: une approche comparative. *Revue Française d'Administration Publique* 76:649-62.

Donabedian, A. 1989. Institutional and professional responsibilities in quality assurance. *Quality Assurance in Health Care* 1(1):3-11.

Hannan, E. L., H. Kilburn, M. Racz., E. Shields, and M. R. Chassin. 1994. Improving the outcomes of coronary artery bypass surgery in New York State. *Journal of the American Medical Association* 271:761-6.

Kazandjian, V.A., P.E. Dans, and L. Sherlis. 1989. What physicians should know about small area variation analysis. *Maryland Medical Journal* 87:477-81.

Kimberly, J. R., and G. de Pouvourville. 1993. Managerial innovation, migration and DRGs. In *The Migration of Managerial Innovation*, edited by J. Kimberly, and G. de Pouvourville G. San Francisco: Jossey Bass.

Lebeer, G. 1997. La violence thérapeutique. *Sciences Sociales et Santé* 15(2):69-96.

McGlynn, E.A. 1997. Six challenges in measuring the quality of health care. *Health Affairs* 16 (3): 7-21.

de Pouvourville, G., J. Andral, and P. Lombrail. Quelles applications pour le Réseau Santé Social ? In *L'informatisation du Cabinet Médical du Futur*, edited by A. Venot, and H. Falcoff. Paris:Springer.

de Pouvourville, G. 1997. Quality of care initiatives in the French context. *International Journal for Quality in Health Care* 9 (3):163-70.

Roper, P. 1989. Shattuck Lecture-Outcome management: a technology of patient experience. *New England Journal of Medicine* 318: 23-5.

Schumacher, D. 1989. *Le case-mix management au quotidien.* Paper presented at Congrés ADAGIO, Paris, 1-2 June 1989.

Starr, P. 1997. Smart technology, stunted policy: Developing health information networks. Health Affairs 16 (3):91-105.

Office of Technology Assessment (U.S. Congress). 1988. *The quality of medical care: Information for consumers.* OTA-H-386. Washington, DC: U.S. Government Printing Office.

Winickoff, R.N., K. L. Coltin, M. M. Morgan, R. C. Buxbaum, and G. O. Barnett. 1984. Improving physician performance through peer comparison feedback. *Medical Care* 22 (6):527-34.

Chapter 3

Quality Management in French Hospitals: From Implicit Concern to Radical Change

Dominique Tonneau

Quality is becoming increasingly important in French hospitals and new management approaches, based on experiences in the United States and the French industrial sector, are being applied (Deming 1982; Harrington 1991; Riveline 1997; Kimberly and Tonneau 1998). Quality is now used as an argument to claim more resources and to justify disagreeable measures. Quality has a new status in health care management, forcing managers and physicians to change their discourse and approach to health care.

Does this mean that in the past quality was never discussed or that nobody cared about it? Certainly not. This chapter aims to show how quality issues were dealt with before the 1990's and how quality, or at least forms of quality, have been the concern of decision-makers for some time. These approaches were, however, not sufficient to consider quality in its entirety. Currently, quality has gained a visibility and an importance, which it did not previously have, and this new management perspective will in all likelihood endure and result in improvements in health status. Although there is a component of "fashion" in the spread of the new quality philosophy, the approach will be an integral part of the evolution of hospital management. Those who use quality on a piecemeal, task-oriented basis, may harm their institutions, and on the other hand, those who understand the commitment involved in a new and global approach to quality as a real management philosophy, will reap substantial benefits.

The perspective developed in this chapter is based upon the author's experience as a researcher and a consultant in management at a research center located at the Ecole des Mines de Paris. Research at this institution uses a combination of theoretical approaches and is conducted in various industries and the public sector. Much of the work has focussed on decision making and control in large organizations in order to understand the role of management tools and procedural obstacles to policy implementation. Hospitals have often been used for these studies, and this chapter is based upon the experience of three decades of investigation in the health sector, either as a consultant to different hospitals (many of them in Paris), or as an advisor to Ministerial Committees (Tonneau et al. 1996; Moisdon and Tonneau 1999).

Based on this experience, I will argue that the term "quality" has been used to refer to attitudes and targets that, at various times, have occupied the thoughts of policy-makers. We shall see that physicians, however, have consistently considered quality, keeping their conclusions to themselves or exposing them only to peer review. Managers have dealt with quality, initially on a quantitative basis, in order to ascertain the level of services required and optimally allocate resources. Government has used quality concepts in its attempts to improve health policy, merge institutions and set the broad guidelines of what can be seen as a form of managed care. The nursing profession has used quality for its own development and to increase its influence in hospitals through the organization of care. Recently, financing institutions began promoting a quality policy that is oriented towards both the individual patient and the population. Difficulties, reluctance and opposition to the promotion of quality are complex issues and it is useful to learn from previous failures and successes as new approaches are developed.

Quality in Medicine

The rapid evolution of medical science can be attributed to our improved understanding of human physiology, the easier dissemination of knowledge, advances in pharmaco-therapeutics and technological breakthroughs in imaging, diagnostics and surgical intervention. These advances have resulted in considerable improvements in the health of populations, at least in industrialized countries. Diseases regarded as common less than a century ago can be easily prevented and treated and the human life span has increased considerably. Not only has medical science increased life expectancy, but it has also improved the quality of life that we can expect as we age.

Physicians in their professional practices keep exploring new ways of improving the service they provide. This is partially motivated by the quest to discover and improve one's reputation among his or her peers. The benefits to patients include the cure of illnesses, decreases in recovery time and morbidity associated with treatment, a wider range of intervention options (such as minimally invasive procedures) and a better quality of life. Medical research requires the objective comparison of new interventions against old (often using controlled trials) and consideration of issues such as quality of life. Consequently, physicians attempt to meet the population's first demand, namely to enjoy a normal life of good quality, for as long as possible. Although this viewpoint is generally accepted, it is worth repeating. This concern with quality has not been obvious to those outside medicine, because it was largely regarded as an internal professional issue.

Medical progress has not been without its problems. As old plagues disappear, new ones arise, such as the range of emerging infectious diseases. Medical progress is largely limited to industrialized countries and communities that can afford high quality care. Inhabitants of less-developed countries often have only limited access to medical resources, and although this question lies in the social rather than medical domain, it will be discussed later in this chapter.

Resource Allocation

As medicine becomes more technologically sophisticated, and therefore more expensive, issues of affordability, accessibility and efficiency inevitably arise. Quality is not only an issue facing individuals, but also confronts health systems and nations. Following W.W.II, quality was considered as a problem of how to spread health facilities throughout France in order to ensure that communities had the best access to the health care. Hospitals were encouraged to expand and keep up with technological progress. This was made possible through a National Insurance system funded by both employer and employee contributions.

By the end of the 1960's, X-ray departments were under pressure to improve facilities and acquire sophisticated imaging technology. Modern technology was expensive and the demand for imaging procedures was growing. X-ray departments were regarded as causing delays in the diagnosis, treatment and discharge of patients, resulting in unnecessary bed occupancy; in some cases, the delay was reported to have been as much as three weeks. The situation became critical and in Paris, where the central hospital administration operates about fifty hospitals, managers were confronted by radiologists, who with the support of clinicians, demanded more machines. It was important to ascertain whether individual hospital requests were justified, which technology should be acquired and to which hospital machines should be allocated. The assistance of Centre de Gestion Scientifique researchers was requested, as they had the required technological and engineering background, experience in management issues, and were familiar with the resource allocation issues. Following 2 years of research at various X-ray departments in Paris which included observation of processes and participants and the collection of quantitative data, the researchers proposed a method of simulating the functioning of a department to calculate equipment and personnel requirements. Radiologists, who had been involved as subjects of the research recommended that the resource allocation methodology be universally applied (Moisdon and Tonneau 1973). The administration granted this request and the researchers conducted a biannual working group meeting where radiologists and chief nurses of the hospital group applied the simulation methods in order to allocate resources.

Our results indicated that although there was an overall lack of radiological equipment, some hospitals were over-equipped (for example, where leading professors had succeeded in having their demands met) and others were severely under-equipped. Resource allocation decisions were also influenced by whether hospitals provided a 24-hours and weekend radiology service. Although the simulations provided a rational approach to the allocation of radiology resources, the final actual distribution did not reflect the results of the studies. In fact, just the opposite occurred, with hospitals that did not lengthen service times getting new equipment and other hospitals, requiring equipment to increase service periods, not receiving an allocation.

In fact, what had occurred demonstrates a common feature in the management of large organizations. The necessity to delegate tasks leads to the splitting of management teams into different departments who do not coordinate activities. Equipment provision was not linked to needs, and problems existed with the allocation of extra staff for after-hours and weekend service. This was connected to inflexible models of staffing and the manipulation of existing rules by various departments. Under these circumstances, management criteria based on quantitative data, were an obstacle to the promotion of quality, although a quality improvement policy was supported by the administration and the medical staff. As resource allocation was not linked to actual service provision, professionals were forced to keep quality as an implicit concern. The allocation of resources was being managed by a centralized administration, splitting the investment amount among disciplines, within disciplines and between hospitals. In such a context, patient concerns could not be taken into account. This policy has now been changed and hospitals are now considered as single units, allowing them to develop projects for the benefit of the patients.

Efficiency, Guidelines and Costs

From the mid-1970s, costs began to concern parties involved in the control of the health system namely, politicians, ministerial administrations, both at national and local levels, and the National Insurance adminstration. Quantitative goals, in terms of facilities, staffing and equipment, had largely been met and there was growing concern about the cost of the health system, particularly hospitals which accounted for over 50% of all expenditure. At this stage, it was decided to consider costs and allocate new resources to departments that could argue that additional resources would decrease their costs. At that time (between about 1975 and 1980), automated and computerized biochemistry and pathology machinery became available, and the Paris hospitals began to face issues previously encountered by X-ray departments.

At an early stage, researchers noted that issues involved in biochemistry and pathology systems were far more complex than those associated with radiology, especially in the determination of equipment and personnel requirements (Boigné, Moisdon and Tonneau 1984). Sophisticated automatic batch testing in chemical pathology and hematology laboratories requires very little staff and provides a wide range of diagnostic information. The availability of numerous tests and rapid results influences the behavior of physicians, who often choose the safest option of ordering the largest possible number of tests, even if some are not directly indicated. It soon became clear that it would be unrealistic to implement the simulation method used for the X-ray departments, and the researchers proposed the use of focus groups, composed of managers from all areas (equipment, personnel, computing services and accountancy), laboratory physicians, technologists, clinicians, engineers, and technicians, who could meet over a longer period, study and discuss the issues and propose new approaches to the resource allocation and personnel problems. Between focus group meetings, the researchers collected and analyzed data to assist in the discussions and tested the validity of different arguments produced by the group. The focus group approach was very constructive, as it allowed people to understand different points of view and take a longer-term view of resource allocation issues. New management tools were designed, including an inventory of all already installed equipment and surveys of how various laboratories were organized.

Stemming from the focus groups, clinicians and laboratory physicians launched a number of studies on the prescribing of tests, what was expected of the results, their transmission and use. Questions asked included:

Should a standardized series of tests be administered on the first day of admission, and would this spare the patient from repeated venipuncture?

How were the results stored in the clinical department, was the physician aware of the last results when he prescribed the next series of tests, and was a longitudinal database available containing all the patient's test results?

Were all tests necessary? In some cases, when test results were kept by the laboratory, nobody claimed them. Patients were often subjected to repeated testing when they moved from one department to another and in some cases tests were carried out although it was known that they had no diagnostic utility.

Could diagnostic test guidelines be drawn up for specific departments or diseases? Particularly, could variations between physician practices for the same disease be reduced using the best available evidence?

Who made decisions as to the diagnostic procedures required for a specific condition and did the clinician collaborate with the laboratory when deciding which tests to order?

The aforementioned questions exposed the nature of the relationship between clinical departments and the laboratories, particularly raising the question of whether the laboratories were merely technical service providers or partners in the investigation of the patient. Although not specifically called quality issues, the problems highlighted in areas such as organizational management, cost-benefit analysis and the relationship between various services within the hospital, forced participants to take a more "global", cross-disciplinary view of patient care.

At first, much analytical data were produced, which assisted both managers and laboratory physicians in better understanding the objectives of the facilities, their primary clients, operations and resource requirements. Thereafter, a dialogue was initiated between laboratory and clinical physicians concerning the most appropriate diagnostic approach. Finally, a series of documents was introduced to collect all the data necessary to understand the operations of the laboratories, and to provide the information needed by the administration to allocate resources. The group provided the documentary evidence to the administration in order to facilitate the annual allocation process. Although the administration professed interest in the methodology, they did not participate, claiming that they did not have the time for a task, which they regarded as outside the scope of their responsibilities.

Furthermore, as in the example of the X-ray departments, the parameters used to allocate resources had undesirable consequences. The cost-allocation procedure resulted in well-equipped laboratories being the first to get more new equipment. As in the case of radiology, a well meaning plan for equitable resource allocation resulted in a misallocation of resources due to a lack of support from management, which continued to use inappropriate criteria. Despite the fact that the work indicated a path towards quality in patient care, managerial constraints forced physicians to use "traditional" strategies such as increasing throughput, to gain further resources.

The Nursing Profession and Quality of Care

Nurses in France do not have a similar status to nurses in the United States, United Kingdom, or Canada. They are employed by individual hospitals, and as almost all responsibility for patient care rests with physicians, nurses have little power on the ward. In university hospitals, department heads are also university professors and as such, are appointed for life[1]. Professors are responsible for one or several wards and their staffing. Although nominally, nurses fall under a chief nurse in the hospital administration, nothing in a department can be changed without the professor's consent. During the 1980's, the situation of nurses changed. Nurses, increasingly aware of the American philosophy of nursing demanded an expanded role in patient care. In particular, they sought to be considered as practitioners of nursing care, and not merely as subordinates implementing doctors' prescriptions. Using current advances in nursing science, especially holistic approaches to patient care, nurses sought to promote their role in the health system. They also used tools and procedures, including nursing diagnosis, the nursing file and nursing care research, to support their position. Although nurses' claims were certainly valid, they provoked negative reactions from some doctors, who saw this behavior as a negation of medical leadership and as an attempt to usurp their power in the hospital.

There was, for example, resistance to the use of the nursing file that contained nursing care information about the patient. The nursing file aims to rationalize patient management data and provide a simple, standardized and verifiable plan for patient care. Nurses who promoted this new concept were better trained and felt that the nursing plan was one way of finally obtaining some acknowledgment from physicians. It should have been relatively easy to introduce the new system, but resistance came from both physicians and nurses. Physicians thought that the nurses wanted to take over their responsibilities and some nurses were suspicious of the increased paperwork and the fact that this was an externally developed methodology imposed on their daily activities. Eventually, a decree from the Ministry of Health was necessary to force every hospital to use nursing files and after a few years, this procedure was fully accepted.

Nurses also tried to promote a policy of quality within their departments, focusing on their own working conditions. As mentioned, department heads have near absolute control and their interests lie mainly in the medical condition of the patients and not in the working conditions of nurses. As little changed concerning their workload, schedules, security and training, nurses went on strike in 1988 and held nationwide demonstrations, demanding reform and proper acknowledgment of their role. This action resulted in some subsidies to finance improved working conditions, and hospitals were permitted to ask for co-financing to deal with nurses' problems.

Does all this activity mean that nurses have promoted quality within hospitals? Although not involved in explicit quality issues, nurses have promoted a concern about quality, especially in the area of individual patient care. Quality was used by nurses, both as an objective and as a way of supporting their position in the debate with physicians. Progress towards quality was made within organizations at an "implicit" level, as everything was influenced by the needs and practices of doctors. The argument over the rights of nurses did, however, evoke the quality issue and force parties to think about care in a more "global" manner. On the other hand, the use of quality in arguments over professional status can have a negative result, if strong opposition is provoked from one or other party.

Budgeting and Quality Measurement

As costs in the French health system continued to rise and the economic situation worsened, with growing unemployment, it became increasingly difficult to ensure a balance between health system expenditure and income provided by payroll—based social insurance. Despite managerial incentives to control expenditures and attempts to avoid the inappropriate acquisition of expensive capital equipment, costs continued to rise. The inflationary trend in health sector expenditure was thought to represent a structural problem in the financing system and to require radical correction (Mossé 1998).

Prior to 1982, each hospital calculated an annual per-diem rate, by dividing gross expenses by the number of patient days[2]. On this basis, the hospital negotiated the following year's per-diem rates with the local supervising body and when the agreement was reached, applied these rates to the bills that were sent to the National Insurance for payment. The National Insurance had no real influence over the amount that they would be charged by individual hospitals, and if a hospital had an annual deficit, this was incorporated into the following year's charges for payment by the National Insurance. The lack of an incentive to contain costs at a hospital level resulted in a decision in 1983 by the Ministry of Health to revise the payment procedure. Each hospital was granted a budget at the beginning of the year and would have to operate within this budget, irrespective of the level of service provided. Hospitals could only spend the amount allocated by the National Insurance. Budgets were simply calculated by increasing the previous year's allocation with a standard increment. Of course, the local supervising bodies could always allow for some margin based on an audit of a particular hospital, but the procedure generally was as described. This situation continued for about ten years, and each year the application of a standard rate to all hospitals increased the inequality between those hospitals that had large allocations in 1983, and those that had smaller initial allocations. The fixed budgeting system was accused of hampering hospitals' ability to develop new activities, or to adjust to changes in the health care needs of local communities. The AIDS epidemic, for instance, made it necessary to grant special budgets to specific hospitals.

For this reason, a new management tool sought to adjust budgets using activity parameters rather than historical expenditures. The tool, imported from the United States, was the DRG (Diagnosis Related Groups) system, called PMSI in France. It took approximately ten years to adapt the DRG system to French conditions, whereafter it was rapidly implemented. Currently all hospitals have to measure their case mix using DRGs following a standardized procedure. Standard costs are applied to each hospital's case-mix, in order to determine the budget that it should receive, if the case-mix was treated at the standard cost. Some hospitals appeared to be over-budget and some operated well under-budget. Supervising bodies now have a more adequate tool to allocate the budgets appropriately and DRG-identified budget inequalities between regions and hospitals, are now gradually being corrected.

Since the "quantity" argument has been clarified using DRGs and activity measures (ISA), quality remains the only argument available to managers and physicians to justify increases in budget and claim more resources. Similarly, as costs are never a very popular justification, authorities also invoke quality when they want to close part of, or an entire hospital. For instance, quality and security for patients have been at the core of the arguments used when it was decided to close a number of maternity hospitals[3]. Unfortunately, these quality claims were never supported by any serious study, making quality a mere argument invoked when required, and not supported by available facts.

The 1996 "Juppé plan" created a national Accreditation Agency in charge of the evaluation of quality in hospitals, a procedure similar to that already in use in the United States and the United Kingdom. It is still too soon to assess what the results of the accreditation initiative will be, but it will probably assist in making quality the main focus of managers and doctors in the coming years. Physicians are working intensely to introduce guidelines for good practice, and managers are working on quality improvement related to hospital reception and registration areas and logistics. Undoubtedly, the organization of hospital departments is going to be a real issue when audits are conducted by the Accreditation Agency. It is likely that these audits will support nurses' procedural recommendations for departmental management. The possibility exists that as the accreditation procedure may look at quality in more general terms, and networks may be built up between hospitals and primary care physicians to provide a better service.

It seems reasonable to claim that quality has finally come out into the open and is an important topic in the health sector (Engel, Moisdon and Tonneau 1992). What lessons can we learn from this history of the slow "introduction" of quality? Is quality likely to remain a temporary management fad or will it become a real and long-term management technique?

Towards "Genuine" Quality Management?

Hospitals in France are regarded as autonomous, but depend on public supervisory bodies for authorization to increase the number of beds, acquire specific equipment and to set prices charged to the National Insurance. Although a quality improvement intervention may be a well thought out answer to a particular problem and represent shared concerns, each stakeholder operates according to a certain internal logic and uncomplicated cooperation is difficult. An example of this has been the coordination of emergency services in Paris (Bolus 1997; Gagneux et al. 1998). General interest does not always yield a common will to promote a quality solution. This explains why quality often remains an implicit internal concern or manifests itself as part of professionals' strategies. Who then should drive an explicit quality strategy and enforce it? From the various examples that have been briefly described, a few lessons can be learned:

Medical science has always been concerned with quality, even if this concern was not explicit. Improvements in diagnosis, therapeutics and the control of infectious diseases have increased life expectancy[4] and made those added years more comfortable. All these efforts can be broadly classified as a search for quality.

As the social financing of medicine has increased, it has resulted in a need to control the resources allocated. Economists, managers, sociologists and politicians, rather than only physicians, have taken a growing interest in these issues. The range of disciplines has resulted in new dimensions of quality being explored, such as best available practices, equity in the allocation of resources, equal access to health services, the relevance of tests or treatments and patient-centered approaches.

Cost-containment concerns, although quite logical for those balancing a National Insurance budget, have been interpreted by others as a thinly disguised argument for reducing services or closing facilities. Quality has acquired the dubious reputation of being a weapon to close facilities, at the very same time as it is proposed as an innovative management approach.

The quality approach has to overcome the barriers within current management procedures (Neuville 1996; Fontaine et al. 1997). Management tools reflect the nature of an organization, its characteristics and timetables. In the real world, management tools tend to limit expectations and demands for change until the discrepancy between the necessity to produce, serve or act is so great as to demand action. At this stage, new tools must be designed to give a more adequate representation of reality.

Health professionals try to ensure that their individual needs get priority and use quality to attain their objectives. This behavior is no surprise to those who study organizations. Directly fighting this attitude is not helpful and it is more important to use self-interest for the purpose of achieving a desired change. This means that quality cannot be a concern solely of managers or regulators, but should be rooted in the concerns of the professionals, their representative bodies, and institutions.

Quality must not become a weapon in the hands of regulators or insurance companies to judge and control either hospitals or physicians. Quality assessment should be based on a shared evaluation of practices, which means both shared knowledge and shared quality criteria[5] .

Quality demands a radical change in the way we consider the health system and health outcomes (de Kervasdoué 1999). A new style of quality oriented management requires criteria to assess the level of quality, methods to increase physician involvement in the running of their departments and hospitals and an increased focus on the patient. Although we are seeing a trend towards the aforementioned manifestations of quality, it would be presumptuous to say that quality management is already an integral part of the French hospital system. Stakeholders, particularly physicians, are not yet completely convinced that quality management can bring them anything, other than financial and practice constraints. Managers are enmeshed in day-to-day financial issues and cannot take a global view of the "chain of patient care" when considering the problems faced by a particular hospital.

A few elements of quality are taking shape. Guidelines are being edited by physicians, consensus conferences are being held to improve diagnosis and therapy, practice guidelines are being issued by the national insurer and continuous education is being promoted. Supervisory bodies and the National Insurance are trying to coordinate services and protect the interests of the patient. As yet, no standardized measures of quality exist. A magazine which published a comparison between hospitals based on "quality criteria" (for surgical departments, this was the number of deaths and the number of people coming for treatment from outside the county) evoked substantial protest from many quarters. Hospitals and physicians were outraged at the idea of being evaluated and managers and economists criticized the inappropriate evaluation criteria.

There is always a danger that any new approach will become too "dogmatic". Could that be the case with quality? Some people see this as a potential problem, while others think that quality will just be another transitory management fashion. There is certainly a "fashion effect" manifest in the spread of a doctrine already prevailing in private companies, or in other industrialized countries. This however does not invalidate the concept of quality. We have seen how quality approaches have been hampered by the misguided logic of stakeholders, the misuse of some management tools and a lack of financial incentives. Today however, we find real drivers, both financial (as an argument for a larger budget), and procedural (to derive advantage from accreditation) of quality in health care. Various parties can satisfy their own interests by joining forces to meet the new targets and implement a quality policy.

Quality is a growing topic of discussion among patients, who are demanding more information and quantifiable results. Hospitals are being held accountable for treatment decisions and compared, based on outcomes. Although the need for objective evaluation of institutional quality is urgent, quality standards should not be too inflexible or unattainably high. Hospitals operate in rapidly changing environments and innovation requires a certain degree of flexibility.

Quality cannot be left to economists or managers. It must include physicians. Nothing is worse than the misuse of quality simply as an argument to justify essentially economic decisions such as budget cuts or the refusal to purchase equipment. The temptation to invoke quality in this way can only be offset by a long-term effort involving all relevant stakeholders to develop a global, patient-centered quality.

Quality is currently the subject of extensive reflection and debate. This is an important process, as the improvement of quality remains a noble goal that can inspire and engage all stakeholders to collaborate and develop a global vision of care. Patients, the new health care consumers, no longer blindly accept the notion that quality is an implicit concern of health care professionals. They (and their insurers) are increasingly demanding information and comparative evaluation of costs and results. Physicians and managers have to deal with this concern, not simply using new techniques or procedures, but rather by radically changing their practices and their way of seeing the health system. This new vision will allow all the actors to understand, and derive benefit from the multi-faceted quality revolution in health care.

Notes

[1] Recently, this system was changed and nominations are now only valid for 5 years. In reality, at the end of 5 years, professors are automatically re-appointed for the following 5-year period.

[2] There were in fact several per-diem rates, based on each department such as general medicine, intensive care and surgery.

[3] The activity threshold being fixed at 300 births a year.

[4] Medicine has not been the only factor resulting in improved life expectancy. One also needs to consider the role of water supply, sanitation, nutrition, housing and improved living standards.

[5] In France, these criteria still need to be developed.

References

Boigné, J. M., J. C. Moisdon, and D. Tonneau. 1984. For a global approach of biochemistry in hospitals. *Social Science and Medicine* 21(10):1167-76.

Bolus, I. 1998. Revue d'information des anesthésistes réanimateurs. *Assurance Qualité* Novembre:4-9.

Deming, E. 1982. *Quality, productivity, and competitive position*. Massachusetts: MIT Press.

Engel, F., J. C. Moisdon, and D. Tonneau. 1992. Proclaimed or effective constraint? Analysis of the regulation in the French public hospitals system (Contrainte affichée ou contrainte réelle? analyse de la régulation du système hospitalier public). *Sciences Sociales et Santé* 8 (2):11-32.

Fontaine, A., P. Vinceneux, A. F. Pauchet, and C. Catala. 1997. Toward quality improvement in a French hospital: structures and culture. *International Journal for Quality in Health Care* 9(3):177-181.

Gagneux, E., P. Lombrail, H. Pichon, and M. Vichard 1998. *Total quality management: une expérience pratique basée sur une double approche conceptuelle dans un service d'accueil des urgences traumatologiques*. Paper presented at XXIèmes journées des économistes de la santé, Paris.

Harrington, H. J. 1991. *Le coût de la non-qualité*. Paris: Ed. Eyrolles.

de Kervasdoué, J. 1999. *Santé, pour une révolution sans réforme*. Paris: Gallimard.

Kimberly, J. R., and D. Tonneau. 1998. The changing role of hospitals in their local market (Le changement du rôle des hôpitaux dans leur environnement local). *Gestions hospitalières* 379:613-16.

Moisdon, J.C., and D. Tonneau. 1973. Organization and functioning of an X-Ray department (Organisation et fonctionnement d'un service de radiodiagnostic). *Revue Hospitalière de France* 261:539-59.

Moisdon, J.C., and D. Tonneau. 1999. *La démarche gestionnaire à l'hôpital, 1—recherches sur la gestion interne.* Paris: Seli Arslan.

Mossé, P. 1998. La rationalisation des pratiques médicales, entre efficacité et effectivité. *Sciences sociales et santé* 16 (4):35-58.

Neuville, J. 1996. La qualité en question. *Revue française de gestion* Mars-mai: 37-48.

Riveline, C.1977. A new approach to company economics (Esquisse d'une nouvelle économie d'entreprise). *Annales des Mines Paris* 4:7-14.

Tonneau, D., S. Bonhoure, A. M. Gallet, and M. Pepin. 1996. Work organization in medical units (L'organisation du travail dans les services de soins). Paris:Editions ANACT.

Part II. Practices

Chapter 4

Coordination and Patient Care Outcomes

Martin P. Charns, Gary J. Young, Jennifer Daley, Shukri F. Khuri and
William G. Henderson

Growing evidence suggests that patient outcomes are related to how effectively
health care organizations coordinate work responsibilities among their staff.
A number of studies have reported on the relationship between coordination
within patient care units and patient outcomes (Argote 1982; Georgeopoulos
1986). Recent studies of intensive care units indicate that better coordination
among clinical staff is associated with lower mortality (Knaus et al. 1987;
Shortell et al. 1992). Baggs et al. (1992) also reported that a higher level of
collaboration between physicians and nurses was related to better patient
outcomes in intensive care units (ICUs).

The role of coordination in health care organizations is also gaining
increased recognition from quality assessment agencies. For example, the Joint
Commission on the Accreditation of Healthcare Organizations (Joint
Commission) recently added several standards to its hospital accreditation
manual addressing the coordination of patient care. One of these standards
stipulates: "The hospital ensures coordination among the health professionals
and services or settings involved in a patient's care."(Joint Commission on
Accreditation of Healthcare 1989:231) Other accrediting bodies such as the
National Committee on Quality Assurance (NCQA) also have accreditation
standards that emphasize coordination among professional staff in the delivery
of health care services.

Notwithstanding this increased awareness of coordination as a determinant
of patient outcomes, information is lacking on actual practices that can be
used to achieve effective coordination. Previous research has tended to report
statistical relationships between global measures of coordination and patient
outcomes but does not offer specific examples of coordination mechanisms
that organizations have implemented. In this chapter we draw from the

experiences of the National Veterans Affairs Surgical Risk Study (NVASRS) to highlight best practices in the coordination of surgical care.

Surgical services are an excellent setting for studying the role of coordination in patient care delivery. A typical surgical service is comprised of several interdependent units—patient floors, operating room, surgical intensive care unit (SICU), and recovery room—among which patients are transferred during the course of an inpatient stay for surgical care. The interdependency among these units implies a strong need for coordination among surgical staff. Moreover, the provision of surgical care involves the participation of several types of professionals, primarily surgeons, anesthesiologists and nurses. The interdependency among these professional groups also implies an important role for coordination in the provision of surgical care.

The research we discuss in this chapter combines two methodologies to investigate the relationship between coordination and risk-adjusted outcomes. The first is the development of risk adjusted surgical outcomes, as part of the NVASRS (National Veteran's Affairs Surgical Risk Study), an extensive project to provide measures of organizational outcomes. The second is the investigation of coordination within the surgical services that comprised the sites for the study. In investigating coordination, we administered a survey to chiefs of the surgical services to obtain background information, conducted in-depth site visits to a sample of 20 sites, and administered a survey to surgical staff in 44 VA surgical services[1].

The National Veterans Affairs Surgical Risk Study

In 1991, the Department of Veterans Affairs launched the National Veterans Affairs Surgical Risk Study (NVASRS). The purpose of the NVASRS is to foster continuous quality improvement in surgical care. The study consists of two major components: (1) the development and validation of a methodology for adjusting patient outcomes to account for differences in the preoperative risk of surgical patients, and (2) the identification of best clinical and management practices for providing surgical care. The surgical services of 44 Department of Veterans Affairs (VA) hospitals participated in the first phase of the study. Each participating surgical service was affiliated with a medical school and was involved in graduate medical education in surgery. Most of the attending surgeons and anesthesiologists had faculty appointments in the affiliated medical school and typically practiced in one or more affiliated hospitals in addition to the VA hospital. All of the study hospitals, as part of the VA system, followed common personnel and fiscal policies. However, these hospitals also had substantial discretion in terms of how they organized and managed patient care activities.

We have discussed the development of validity of the risk-adjustment methods elsewhere (Khuri et al. 1995). In brief, during the first phase of the study, detailed clinical and outcome data were collected prospectively at the 44 participating surgical services between October 1, 1991 and December 31, 1993, a 27-month period. All patients included in the study underwent a major surgical procedure as defined by the use of general, spinal, or epidural anesthesia.

Surgical procedures with very low observed mortality or postoperative morbidity rates were excluded (for example, vascular shunt revision, diagnostic endoscopy, simple incision and drainage of skin abscesses). Operations were collected in eight surgical subspecialties: general surgery, thoracic surgery, peripheral vascular surgery, neurosurgery, orthopaedics, urology, otolaryngology, and plastic surgery. Cardiac surgery information was collected but was analyzed separately as part of the Continuous Quality Improvement in Cardiac Surgery program based at the Denver VAMC (Grover, Hammermeister and Burchfiel 1990; Grover et al. 1993; Grover et al. 1994; Hammermeister et al. 1990; Hammermeister et al. 1994).

Patients' clinical risk factors, intraoperative information, and 30-day postoperative outcomes were collected prospectively on 87,078 surgical procedures. Postoperative outcomes included both mortality and 21 predefined morbidities occurring in the 30 days after the index operation. Preoperative clinical risk factors (total factors = 67), preoperative laboratory results (total results = 17), and intraoperative variables such as the Common Procedural Terminology (CPT-4) code (there were 16 total variables) of the principal operative procedure were noted, as were other associated operative procedures and total operative time.

We used the preoperative variables to develop risk-adjustment models for mortality and postoperative morbidity. Logistic regression was used for surgical mortality which was measured as whether the patient died within 30 days of the index surgical procedure. Logistic regression was also used to model postoperative morbidity, defined as the presence of one or more of the 21 predefined morbidities occurring in the 30 days postoperatively. To account for the underlying risk of the surgical procedure independent of patient risk, we used the ratings of complexity of each of the CPT-4 codes in the data set by panels of Veterans Administration surgical sub-specialists. The panelists rated the complexity of each CPT-4 code on a scale from 1 to 5. The surgical panel ratings were highly correlated with the Resource Based Relative Value Scale weighting scales ($r = 0.76$ for all operations; $p = 0.0001$) (Hsiao et al. 1988a; Hsiao et al. 1988b).

The mortality risk-adjustment model for all operations had 34 patient risk factors and had a c-index of 0.89. Leading predictor variables for all operations included preoperative serum albumin level, American Society of Anesthesia class, emergency scheduling of the operation, the presence of disseminated cancer, age, a blood urea nitrogen > 40 mg/dL, the do-not-resuscitate status of the patient before operation, platelet count $\leq$ 150,000/mL, weight loss > 10% in the 6months before operation, and an elevated serum glutamic oxaloacetic transaminase level. (Khuri et al. 1995).

The postoperative morbidity model for all operations had 18 patient risk factors and a c-index of 0.78. The leading predictor variables for postoperative morbidity were similar, but not identical, to those for the mortality models and included preoperative serum albumin, American Society of Anesthesia class, the complexity score of the principal operation, emergency scheduling of the operation, the patient's functional status before the operation, use of ventilation before operation, wound infection before operation, a history of chronic obstructive pulmonary disease, and a hematocrit $\leq$ 38% (Grover, Hammermeister, and Burchfield 1990).

The logistic regression models were used to estimate the probability of death or postoperative morbidity for each patient. The expected mortality rate for each VAMC surgical service was calculated by summing the probabilities of death for each of its cases. The observed VAMC mortality rate was then compared with the expected VAMC mortality rate in the form of an observed-to-expected ratio (O/E ratio). A similar O/E ratio was calculated for postoperative morbidity. Among the 44 surgical services the ratios ranged between .49 and 1.53 for mortality, and between .49 and 1.46 for morbidity. Services with O/E ratios less than 1.0 have lower than expected rates of adverse outcomes, and those greater than 1.0 have higher than expected rates.

Statistical outliers from the average O/E ratio of 1.0 were calculated using an exact method to compute the confidence interval for a binomial proportion. Confidence intervals that did not include 1.0 indicated high or low outlier hospitals. The O/E ratios were kept in strict confidence for the duration of the study. Of the 44 VAMCs, 13 were statistical outliers for mortality at the 90% confidence interval (6 high and 7 low), and 20 were statistical outliers for postoperative morbidity at a 99% confidence interval (8 high and 12 low).

Coordination Conceptual Framework

Coordination has been defined as the conscious activity of assembling and synchronizing differentiated work efforts so that they function harmoniously in attainment of organizational objectives (Haimann, Scott, and Connor 1978). Several typologies have been developed to study coordination. In this study, we were guided by a well-developed typology (Longest and Klingersmith 1994; March and Simon 1958; Mintzberg 1979) that has previously been applied to health care organizations (Alt-White, Charns, and Strayer 1983; Argote 1982; Becker, Shortell, and Neuhauser 1980; Charns and Lockhart 1994; Charns and Schaefer 1983). In this typology, coordination mechanisms are categorized into two major groups: *programming* (or standardized) and *feedback* (or personal) methods. Programming approaches seek to clarify work responsibilities and activities in advance of the performance of the work, as well as specify the outputs of the work process and the skills required to perform the work.

Programming Approaches

Programming approaches are most effective when the work requirements are well understood and predictable. Two major types of programming are:

Standardization of work is the use of rules, regulations, schedules, plans, procedures, policies, and protocols to specify the activities to be performed. It also includes specification of the form of intermediate outcomes of work as they are passed from one job to another and of the final products or services.

Standardization of skills is the specification of the skills or information required to perform work. Often this is achieved through specification of minimum levels and types of education, certification as evidence of meeting minimum qualifications, or orientation and other on-the-job training.

Programming approaches are relatively efficient to use, as they require little time for personal interaction. They work well for routine work. In situations of high uncertainty, however, programming approaches alone cannot provide the needed coordination. Exchange of information and feedback among staff are needed for adapting to unforeseen circumstances or events.

Feedback Approaches

Feedback mechanisms, which facilitate the transfer of information in unfamiliar situations, include:

Supervision is the basis for coordination through an organization's hierarchy. It is the exchange of information between two people, one of whom is responsible for the work of the other.

Peer interaction is the exchange of information about work performance between or among people who are not in a hierarchical relationship, such as between two nurses or between a physician and a nurse. Peer interaction can occur in the context of a one-to-one discussion or a group meeting such as a mortality and morbidity conference.

Feedback approaches to coordination are more time consuming and require more effort than programming approaches. However, organization theory suggests that feedback approaches are needed in situations characterized by high levels of uncertainty. In general, healthcare organizations face relatively unpredictable or uncertain work requirements that also entail high degrees of staff interdependencies (Charns and Schaefer 1983; Flood 1994). A major source of this uncertainty is the variability among patients in response to medical interventions. Thus, patient care processes cannot be completely standardized. High interdependencies exist because the complexity of patient care requires high levels of input from a variety of staff in various clinical specialties (Charns and Schaefer 1983). Based on these characteristics of surgical care, we hypothesized that surgical services with better than expected patient outcomes used feedback approaches to a greater extent than services with worse than expected outcomes.

A longstanding debate in the healthcare management literature, however, is whether programming impedes or facilitates good patient care (Becker, Shortell and Neuhauser 1980; Flood 1994). Some have argued that programming approaches to coordination constrain healthcare professionals from responding to the dynamic requirements of their work. Physician resistance to clinical practice guidelines is an example of this long-standing sentiment (Kapp 1990). Others contend that programming approaches can support feedback if they are used to coordinate routine work, characterized by relatively little uncertainty. This use of programming will free up resources—including the time and attention of healthcare professionals—to be used to coordinate more complex and uncertain work though feedback approaches. Charns and Schaefer (1983) suggest that optimum coordination is achieved in healthcare organizations when both programming and feedback are used to their greatest extent. This view is also consistent with the growing literature on patient safety. That literature suggests combining systems, similar in concept to "programming approaches," and communication, an important element in feedback approaches.

We used this typology of programming and feedback approaches to coordination to address how academically affiliated surgical services coordinate three primary work activities: general administration, direct provision of patient care, and graduate medical education of surgical residents. We focused on these work activities because our preliminary interviews with chiefs of surgery suggested that each work activity is associated with a unique set of challenges for coordinating the work of surgical staff. General administration comprised such activities as developing an organization structure for the surgical service, formulating budgets, monitoring the staff's performance, managing relationships between the surgical service and other parts of the medical center, and obtaining resources. Direct patient care consisted of the actual delivery of clinical services to patients. Graduate medical education referred to the oversight and training of surgical residents. The application of the coordination typology to these three primary work activities provided the study's conceptual framework.

Site Visits

We conducted in-depth site visits to 20 of the 44 surgical services that, based on risk-adjusted mortality and morbidity ratios, were either high or low outliers in terms of surgical outcomes. The site visits were used to collect detailed data about the coordination practices of the 20 surgical services and were used to address two questions:

Are low outliers and high outliers distinguished by the number and variety of coordination practices they use?

What are some best practices for coordinating surgical care?

Study Method

We selected the 20 services to represent each end of the distribution of the risk-adjusted mortality and morbidity ratios. Specifically, low outliers consisted of those surgical services that had either one of the five lowest O/E mortality ratios or one of the five lowest O/E morbidity ratios. High outliers consisted of those surgical services that had either one of the five highest O/E mortality ratios or one of the five highest O/E morbidity ratios. One surgical service met two of the selection criteria: it had one of the five lowest mortality ratios and one of the five lowest morbidity ratios. We included this surgical service in the study because of its mortality status and selected a sixth service to replace it as a morbidity outlier. All selected surgical services were statistical outliers for either mortality or morbidity.

Table 1 presents descriptive data on the low and high outliers participating in the study. High outliers had on average mortality and morbidity ratios that were approximately 40 percent higher than those of the low outliers. While low outliers had a larger number of surgical beds than high outliers on average, the two groups are comparable with respect to the volume of major surgical operations they perform.

Each site visit was conducted by a three-member team consisting of a senior surgeon, a surgical nurse with clinical and management experience in postoperative intensive care, and a member of the research team. Ten surgeons, five nurses, and four members of the research team participated in the site visits. The surgeons and surgical nurses were each selected from among the 44 VA hospitals participating in the NVASRS. Site visits to each surgical service lasted 2 days and involved individual and group interviews with surgical staff. Individual interviews were conducted with the chief of surgery, chief of anesthesia, senior nurse responsible for the surgical service, chief of staff, chief of medicine, a chief resident, and the person responsible for quality assurance on the surgical service. Group interviews were conducted with staff surgeons, nurse managers responsible for the operating room and surgical intensive care unit, nurse managers responsible for the patient care floors, and an interdisciplinary group of surgeons, anesthesiologists, nurses, and clinical support staff (such as ward clerks). In addition to the on-site interviews, the site visit team attended "walk rounds" in the surgical intensive care unit and toured the entire surgical service. Both the site visit team members and the staff at the 20 participating surgical services were blinded to the outlier status of the services during the site visits.

Measurement	Low outliers (n=10)	High outliers (n=10)
Risk-adjusted mortality † O/E ratio	86 (.25)	1.21 (.22)
Risk-adjusted morbidity † O/E ratio	.83 (.22)	1.16 (.19)
Total number of hospital beds	257 (160)	244 (140)
Total number of surgical beds	125 (69)	92 (26)
Annual number of major inpatient surgical operations	1908 (452)	1812 (427)

*Standard deviation in parenthesis.
†Difference between high and low outliers is statistically significant (p<.01).

Table 1. Descriptive Data on High and Low Outliers

All site visits were conducted in accordance with a uniform set of interview protocols. We developed these interview protocols on the basis of the previously discussed conceptual framework that focuses on the nature and effectiveness of coordination practices in the areas of general administration, direct patient care, and graduate medical education.

Site Visit Initial Findings

We first compared the assessment of the outlier status of the sites as judged by the site visit teams, to the outlier status based upon the risk adjusted outcomes. These results are shown in Table 2.

		Site Visitors' Ratings	
		High	Low
Clinical Model Outlier Status	**High**	9	1
	Low	2	8
	Total	11	9

Table 2. Comparison of Site Visitors' Ratings and Risk Adjustment Model Outlier Status for 20 Surgical services

The site visitors correctly identified the outlier status of 17 of the 20 surgical services. Percent exact agreement was 85% (p< 0.001); the kappa statistic was 0.7. They correctly identified nine of the mortality-outlier sites and eight of the postoperative morbidity outliers. They incorrectly identified one low-mortality outlier as a high outlier. For the two other sites, one site visit team incorrectly identified a high-morbidity outlier as a low outlier, and another team incorrectly identified a low-morbidity outlier as a high outlier. The site visitors were not able to identify whether the sites were outliers for mortality as opposed to postoperative morbidity.

Survey of Surgical Staff

To obtain an additional perspective on coordination to augment our site visits, we developed, distributed and analyzed a survey of staff in the surgical services. The survey was based on the same theoretical framework as was used in the site visits and focused on methods of coordination, and perceived quality of care.

Study Method

Sample

The study sample consisted of all 44 surgical services participating in the NVASRS, those in the largest hospitals in the VA healthcare system.

Measures

To obtain information on coordination and on perceived quality, we surveyed three types of surgical staff: attending surgeons, attending anesthesiologists, and nurses. We did not include residents in the survey because, given their rotation among several hospitals, it was difficult to determine when they had sufficient experience at a participating surgical service to provide meaningful information about its coordination practices or quality. To ensure that the survey and clinical outcomes data were contemporaneous, we conducted the staff survey to coincide with phase two of the NVASRS, which occurred between January 1, 1994 and August 31, 1995. The survey was conducted between February 1995 and July 1995.

The survey was mailed to each respondent through the internal mail system of the participating hospitals. Two mailings were conducted. A total of 7,364 surveys were returned, yielding a response rate of 73.2 percent. 2,555 surgeons (response rate 70.9 percent), 467 anesthesiologists (73.0 percent), and 4,342 nurses (74.3 percent) responded. These response rates compare favorably with previous surveys of physicians and nurses that are designed to collect information on management practices (Shortell et al. 1991). Because the surgical service is the unit of analysis for the study, we aggregated responses of individuals. This process and the validity of resulting measures are discussed below.

Clinical Outcomes

Risk adjusted measures of morbidity and mortality came from the second phase of the NVASRS. During phase two, approximately 60,000 operations performed at the 44 study sites were included in the risk adjustment process.

Perceived Quality of Care

To measure perceptions of quality of care, we adopted an existing instrument (Charns et al 1980; Mitchell et al. 1989) that was used previously to assess patient care quality in critical care units and also in general inpatient care units. These earlier studies support the reliability and validity of the instrument. The items ask respondents how effectively various patient care activities are carried out. For example, respondents are asked about the extent to which patient transfers and discharges are handled effectively; the extent to which staff are aware of patients' progress; and the extent to which poor planning and communication lead to mistakes in care. We changed the wording of some items to make them more meaningful to surgical staff. Chronbach's alpha for the instrument was 0.85.

Coordination Approaches
Each item of the questionnaire corresponded conceptually either to coordination based on programming (for example, protocols, pathways, treatment plans), coordination based on group feedback (for example, interdisciplinary rounds, conferences), or coordination based on personal discussion (for example, discussion between two nurses, discussion between a physician and a nurse). Because certain coordination approaches are not relevant to all three professional groups, we developed slightly modified versions of the instrument for surgeons, anesthesiologists and nurses. For example, only nurses were asked about shift reports.

Using a 5-point scale, respondents indicated to what extent each coordination item provided them with information for performing their work. For each respondent we aggregated the responses for individual items, weighting items equally, into two scales: programming and feedback. We then averaged respondents' scale scores to derive scale scores for each professional group. We then aggregated the scores of the three professional groups into scores for the surgical service. As Shortell et al. (1994) did in their study of ICUs, we gave equal weight to the responses from the professional groups. This reflects our desire to capture the pattern of coordination that emerges from all three professional groups working toward the common goal of providing effective care. Had we just aggregated all individual responses directly to the level of the surgical service, the unequal number of respondents in the three groups would have given unequal weight to the different professional groups.

After completing the data aggregation, each surgical service had separate scores for each of the coordination approaches and the perceived quality variable. To test the study's hypothesis concerning patterns of coordination and surgical outcomes, we assigned each surgical service to one of three groups based on its combination of scores on the programming and feedback variables. We collapsed the surgical services into one of three groups rather than use the coordination variables in continuous form primarily, because our site visit observations suggested that very different patterns of coordination characterized the surgical services. In other words, we saw them differing more in kind than degree.

Surgical services scoring above the median on both programming and feedback were assigned to the "high coordination" group. Those scoring below the median on both variables were assigned to the "low coordination" group. The remaining surgical services were assigned to the "intermediate coordination" group. These sites were either above the median on programming and below the median on feedback or below the median on programming and above the median on feedback. From our site visits, we had no basis for distinguishing between these two intermediate patterns of coordination in terms of their likely effects on clinical outcomes.

Structural Characteristics
Previous research points to several structural characteristics that potentially are related to clinical outcomes. To control for possible relationships between structural characteristics and outcomes, we accounted for differences among the sites with regard to technological availability, teaching activity and size. Data for measuring these characteristics were obtained from a questionnaire completed by the chief of surgery in each site.

Results
We first examined correlations among individual variables. Descriptive data and zero-order correlations are presented in Table 3. As seen in the table, a relatively high positive correlation exists between programming and feedback. This result suggests that programming and feedback do not necessarily substitute for each other, as has been suggested in prior research (Van De Ven, Delbecq, and Koenig 1976), but may vary together. The correlation of mortality and morbidity rates is positive but not statistically significant. This is consistent with research by Silber et al. (1992), who also reported non-significant correlation between these two types of clinical outcomes. The available

evidence suggests that factors in hospitals associated with surgical morbidity are somewhat different than those associated with surgical mortality. Perceived quality is negatively correlated with each clinical outcome variable, but these correlations are not significant. This suggests that perceived quality is a limited proxy for quality of care. Both programming and feedback are positively and significantly correlated with perceived quality of care.

Both programming and feedback are correlated with each of the clinical outcome variables in the expected direction (i.e., negatively), but these correlations are not statistically significant. This suggests that neither coordination approach independently has a significant effect on clinical outcomes.

We next performed a multiple regression analysis to examine the effects of the different patterns of coordination with respect to morbidity, mortality and perceived quality, while controlling for the structural characteristics. Dummy variables were used to represent the low- and intermediate-coordination groups, and the high-coordination group was used as the reference group. The regression results are shown in Table 4. In the mortality analysis, contrary to our expectations, the high-coordination group does not have significantly lower mortality than either the low- or intermediate-coordination group. In the morbidity analysis, the coefficient for the low-coordination group is positive and significant, indicating that the low-coordination group has a significantly higher morbidity O/E ratio than the high coordination group. The coefficient for the intermediate-coordination group is positive but not statistically significant. The results of the regression analysis for perceived quality is consistent with what was expected. The coefficients for the low- and intermediate-coordination groups are negative and significant, indicating that the high coordination group has the highest perceived quality of the three groups of surgical services.

	Mean	s.d.*	Range	1	2	3	4
O/E Mortality Ratio	1.02	0.28	0.53– 2.15	–			
O/E Morbidity Ratio	1.05	0.28	0.49– 1.72	0.24	–		
Perceived Quality	3.41	0.12	3.11– 3.69	–0.15	–0.24	–	
Feedback	2.77	0.15	2.38– 3.12	–0.08	–0.18	0.36	–
Programming	2.37	0.19	2.03– 2.83	–0.03	–0.12	0.28	0.51
Technological Availability	75.68	12.69	41.67– 95.83	–0.18	–0.03	0.06	0.01
Teaching Intensity	0.16	0.07	0.09– 0.44	0.09	0.11	0.10	0.12
Size (beds)	104.40	40.90	47– 216	–0.12	–0.19	–0.15	0.07

*Standard deviation

Table 3. Descriptive Data and Zero-Order Correlations for Study Variables

Predictor Variables	O/E Mortality Ratio			O/E Morbidity Ratio			Perceived Quality		
	B	(s.e.)	p	B	(s.e.)	p	B	(s.e.)	p
Constant	1.21	.284	.01	1.066	.267	.01	3.44	.121	.01
Technological Availability	−.005	.004	.19	−.002	.003	.60	.001	.001	.42
Teaching Intensity	.791	.693	.26	.992	.652	.14	−.043	.297	.89
Size (Beds)	−.054	.110	.63	−.171	.103	.11	−.053	.047	.26
Low-coordination Group	.131	.114	.24	.286	.107	.01	−.080	.042	.09
Intermediate-Coordination Group	.137	.197	.21	.111	.101	.28	−.097	.046	.04
R^2	.13			.20			.16		
n	44			44			44		

Table 4. Results from Multiple Regression Analysis

Best practices

Given the findings from the site visits and the staff survey, we wanted to identify management and organizational factors that differentiated the low and high outlier surgical services. To identify these differences, we analyzed the content of the field notes from each site visit. The key findings and representative examples are provided below. The findings are organized by the three work activities forming the study's conceptual framework: general administration, direct patient care, and graduate medical education. The findings reflect patterns of coordination practices that, based on the site visit data, appear to distinguish high and low outliers. Each finding does not apply to every surgical service studied. These are summarized in Table 5.

General Administration

Low outliers were more likely than high outliers to have a variety of coordination mechanisms for addressing both routine and non-routine administrative issues. An important finding is that low outliers used peer interaction very effectively to accomplish the administrative integration of the three primary professional groups—surgeons, anesthesiologists, and nurses. In contrast to high outliers, low outliers were more likely to use peer interaction to ensure that there was adequate input from all three professional groups regarding major administrative decisions affecting surgical care. Peer interaction among low outliers was particularly strong at the level of the surgical service leadership, (i.e., chief of surgery, chief of anesthesia, and nurse managers responsible for the surgical service). Among low outliers, it was common for these leaders to interact through regularly scheduled meetings. The meetings were conducted as "strategy sessions," with discussions typically focusing on future staffing requirements, equipment and space needs, and the tactics for strengthening the interaction of surgical staff.

At low outliers, we found many examples of the surgical service leaders interacting with one another to address administrative issues affecting the overall performance of the surgical service. At two low outliers, the leaders of the surgical service even collaborated in the selection of staff, an activity retained as the exclusive "right" of each professional group in the high outliers. As noted by the chief of surgery of one of these surgical services:

Coordination Approach

		Standardization of work	Standardization of skills	Supervision	Peer interaction
Work Activity	General Administration	Data system for collection of quality Indicators	Staff training to use and interpret data on quality indicators	Chief of surgery profiles attending surgeons and provides feedback on patient outcomes	Leaders of surgical service conduct strategy meetings
	Direct Patient Care	Clinical pathway development and implementation	Clinical nurse specialist in SICU to train staff nurses	Operating room "czar"	Interdisciplinary patient rounds involving physicians and nurses
	Graduate Medical Education	Detailed criteria specifying level and nature of attending oversight of residents	Well-developed orientation program for new residents	Mentoring for residents	Attending surgeons meet regularly to discuss the progress and training of residents

Table 5. Best-Practice Matrix

I have had input in the hiring of every one of the nurse managers. It is not an adversarial relationship between me and nursing service; they never do anything behind my back and I never do anything behind their back.

Although the nurse managers at this surgical service did not have input into the selection of attending surgeons or anesthesiologists, they were involved in the performance assessment of surgical and anesthesia residents.

In contrast to low outliers, high outliers had substantially less peer interaction concerning administrative issues among the three professional groups. When meetings among the leaders of surgery, anesthesia, and nursing did take place, they were more likely to be *ad hoc*, usually in response to a problem or crisis after it had occurred. The absence of such peer interaction at high outliers characterized how the leaders of the surgical service related to one another generally. While at most high outliers we did not hear of any widespread animosity among the leaders of the surgical service, the leaders of these different professional groups often spoke as though they existed independently from each other in caring for surgical patients.

Our interviews with the chiefs of surgery helped provide an understanding of why high outliers had such limited interaction among their professional groups on administrative matters. At two high outliers, the chief remarked that he and the other surgical service leaders were not able to find a time in their schedules to meet regularly. At another high outlier, the chief referred frequently to the importance of "maintaining autonomy and independence of each professional group." Several chiefs, however, commented that they had attempted regular senior leadership meetings but discontinued them after finding two or three initial efforts to be unproductive. This meant that they amounted to little more than what one chief called "gripe sessions." Interestingly, the chiefs of surgery at low outliers noted similar experiences when they first initiated meetings with the leaders of the surgical service. But many of them found that they were able to get past the griping by uniting participants around common problems and issues. Over time, the chiefs found that participants stopped griping and started talking about solutions. One chief described the experience this way:

We had never met regularly as a group before and so people began to use the opportunity to voice their complaints; everyone was pointing their finger at somebody else saying it's your fault. After two meetings, I started writing down complaints and began looking for patterns pointing to common problems. Once I was able to show them that we really were all in the same boat, we began to work together to make improvements.

Low outliers were also more effective than high outliers in using peer interactions to manage relationships with other components of the hospital that provide support to the surgical service. For example, at most low outliers, the chief of surgery frequently met with the chief of medicine (often over lunch) to discuss strategies for improving the timeliness and quality of consultations between the medical and surgical services. The relationship between the chief of surgery and the chief of medicine at high outliers was typically less established. In general, we heard far fewer complaints about the timeliness of medical consults to surgery at low outliers than we did at high outliers. As another example, the chiefs of surgery at low outliers were much more likely than their counterparts at the high outliers to maintain direct communication with a member of the hospital's quality assurance staff. At several low outliers, meetings between the chief of surgery and quality management staff took place at least once a month to allow the chief of surgery to review trends or patterns in surgical outcomes such as mortality, infection rates, and readmissions.

In the area of general administration, another frequently observed difference between low and high outliers was the use of existing supervisory arrangements to monitor and improve quality of care. Supervisors (for example, nurse managers, chiefs of surgery) at low outliers were more likely than those at high outliers to provide their employees with feedback based on objective data about their work and opportunities for improvement. For example, at two low outliers, the chief of surgery maintained outcomes profiles on each attending surgeon and used the data to provide feedback to the attending surgeons on their performance. It was the practice of a chief of surgery at one of these low outliers to disseminate this information monthly and hold meetings individually with each attending surgeon to discuss his or her particular performance.

In addressing administrative issues, low outliers frequently used standardization mechanisms in conjunction with personal coordination approaches. For example, at many of the low outliers, the quality of surgical care was a regular agenda item at meetings of the surgical service leadership. Surgical service leaders were able to focus on this issue objectively because data systems were in place for the collection of quality indicators. The presence of such data systems represents a form of work standardization. Furthermore, opportunities for formal training in using and interpreting quality indicators, which we found to be more common among the low outliers, serve as examples of training and staff development within the area of general administration. Some of the high outliers also had good systems for collecting quality indicators, but the leaders of these services (such as the chief of surgery, chief of anesthesia and chief nurse responsible for the surgical service) were less likely to use the data collaboratively to examine the overall performance of the surgical service.

Direct Patient Care

In terms of direct patient care, low and high outliers were distinguishable not by any obvious differences in the technical competence or dedication of their surgical staff, but rather in the way low outliers coordinated the clinical activities of different professional groups across multiple surgical units. Previous research suggests that greater interdisciplinary collaboration in patient care leads to better patient outcomes (Baggs et al. 1992; Shortell et al. 1992). We too found that low outliers were more likely than high outliers to emphasize peer interaction among professional groups in the delivery of patient care. For example, at many of the low outliers, nurses and surgeons conducted patient rounds together, an activity we did not observe among most high outliers. A surgeon at one of the low outliers commented that interdisciplinary rounds provided opportunities "for a more complete exchange of clinical information."

We found many examples where low outliers found ways to promote and strengthen teamwork among the surgical staff. At two of the low outliers each operating nurse was assigned to a surgical subspecialty and primarily worked with surgeons on that service. Surgeons commented that working with the same nurse on a regular basis "promoted efficiency and trust"; nurses referred to benefits such as "enhanced professionalism" and "stronger skill development." At another low outlier, a surgical intensive care unit (SICU) nurse manager remarked:

Teamwork between nursing and anesthesia here is the best that I have ever experienced, and I have worked at seven hospitals in my career.

Attending anesthesiologists always accompany post-surgical patients to the SICU and, before leaving, provide a full report to either the nurse manager or charge nurse about the patient's clinical status. At many other hospitals anesthesiologists just drop the patients off and return to the O.R.

It is important to note that at high outliers we did not find evidence of hostility toward the idea of interdisciplinary collaboration in patient care. There were simply few mechanisms in place to foster or reinforce such behavior. When compared to low outliers, high outliers were less effective in coordinating the clinical roles and responsibilities of the surgeons, anesthesiologists, and nurses.

Supervision of patient care activities was also substantially better at low outliers than high outliers. We found that many low outliers had created supervisory positions for coordinating surgical activities that typically do not fall within the prerogative of any one professional group. For example, a number of low outliers had what was commonly referred to as "operating room czars," individuals who had ultimate responsibility for coordinating the operating room schedule. The individual serving in this position at one of the low outliers was, by training, a clinical nurse specialist who also had a master's degree in business administration. As the operating room manager, she was the final arbiter among the surgeons, anesthesiologists, and nurses when scheduling conflicts arose. Because she reported directly to the medical center's chief of staff, her authority over scheduling matters was formalized in the medical center's organizational structure. The benefits of having someone in the role were sung by many of the surgical staff with whom we spoke. An attending surgeon commented:

Before [she] took over, there was some degree of confusion and sometimes dissension about whose case would be taken next. She developed a set of scheduling rules for the O.R. and enforces these rules fairly and effectively. Her addition to the O.R. has really helped to reduce unnecessary delays in surgery.

While most of the low outliers relied heavily on personal approaches to coordinate the direct provision of care, they were also further along than high outliers in standardizing clinical activities through the development and implementation of clinical pathways and protocols. Clinical pathways were typically used to coordinate the responsibilities of surgeons and nurses for patient care procedures. At one low outlier, SICU nurses had the authority to extubate patients if certain well-defined criteria were met; otherwise, the decision to extubate was left to the attending surgeon. At another low outlier, a protocol was developed to assist nurses in identifying patients at risk for pressure sores. When at-risk patients were identified, nurses would confer with the attending surgeon to consider appropriate prevention strategies such as ordering a special bed.

Several factors seemed to impede high outliers from moving forward in terms of standardizing clinical activities. At one service, the chief of surgery did not believe in pathways and, consequently, members of the surgical staff considered them a taboo subject. At two high outliers, the resistance came from staff surgeons who found pathways and protocols offensive and a threat to their clinical autonomy. But by and large, for most high outliers the major impediment to standardizing clinical activities was a lack of sustained commitment by the hospital or surgical service leadership to the time and effort required to develop and implement clinical pathways. Low outliers were simply more likely than high outliers to make pathway development a priority. Two examples from our site visits illustrate this point. At one low outlier, we walked into the chief of surgery's office to find his walls adorned with numerous charts depicting completed pathways and pathways under development. The charts identified the individuals responsible for developing each pathway and the expected completion times for preliminary and final products. All pathway teams were chartered by a council consisting of the chief of surgery, chief of anesthesia, and two nurse managers. Each pathway team had an assigned leader who was accountable to the council for the team's results. By contrast, we visited one high outlier where pathway development was "reportedly" under way. However, no central structure had been established to oversee the formation and progress of pathway development teams. We were told that several teams had been assembled to develop pathways but that "scheduling conflicts" among team members had caused them to be "temporarily disbanded."

In the direct provision of patient care, low outliers appeared to be superior to high outliers in the training and development of staff nurses. While no apparent differences existed between low and high outliers regarding the availability and quality of formal nurse continuing education programs, low outliers placed greater emphasis than high outliers on the use of clinical nurse specialists to develop the skills of nurses at the patients' bedside. Almost all low outliers had clinical nurse specialists dedicated to the SICU, whereas several high outliers either never had a clinical nurse specialist or lost the ones they had to staff cutbacks. The absence of this training resource at some of the high outliers was complicated by what appeared to be nursing staff with higher turnover and lower educational levels relative to low outliers. In general, we found that high outliers had more turnover among nursing staff, more frequent use of per diem employees, and were more likely to have nurses (especially in the SICU) with less formal training and education. Indeed, high turnover among nursing staff may be both a cause and consequence of poor coordination. Clearly, a less stable and less formally educated nursing staff would present a barrier to effective coordination and increase the need for training and development efforts. Research also suggests that poor coordination motivates highly qualified nurses to search for positions at other health care organizations (Weisman, Alexander and Chase 1981).

Graduate Medical Education
Low outliers were more successful than high outliers in striking the often-difficult balance between providing surgical residents with clinical experience and ensuring that residents have the appropriate level of oversight. To achieve this balance, low outliers had in place a variety of well-established coordination mechanisms that contributed substantially to residents having a supportive work environment and well-defined roles and responsibilities.

In general, low outliers were more likely than their high outlier counterparts to have training and skills development opportunities to assist residents in their transition to the surgical service. In this respect, differences between low and high outliers can first be observed on July 1 when first-year surgical residents start their rotations. Many of the low outliers had well-developed orientation for these fledgling surgeons covering the physical layout of the service, the availability of technology and other resources, patient care policies and procedures for the service, and the names and telephone extensions of key personnel in the service. By contrast, the orientation for residents at high outliers was typically less comprehensive and not as well organized. Two high outliers did not appear to have any clearly defined orientation program at all for surgical residents. In addition to orientation programs, many low outliers had educational resources in place to support residents in performing clinical tasks. For example, at one low outlier the chief of surgery hired a nurse practitioner to provide educational support to first-year residents in performing routine clinical procedures such as venipuncture and intubation. High outliers were more likely to approach resident training as, in the words of one resident, "a trial by fire process."

In addition, low outliers maintained strong systems of oversight for residents throughout the rotation period. For example, one of the low outliers had a very effective mentoring system in place where each attending surgeon was assigned responsibility for two residents—one senior and one junior. Attending surgeons met regularly with their residents to discuss clinical activities, research developments in surgical care, and personal adjustment issues related to the rotation schedule. It was also apparent that at low outliers residents were more likely to view attending backup surgeon coverage as an accessible and reliable resource than were residents at high outliers. This difference in attitudes seemed rooted in the emphasis on teamwork between attending physicians and residents. Teamwork between attending surgeons and residents was a priority at all the low outliers. This was symbolized at one low outlier by having outside each patient's room, the names of both his or her attending surgeon and the resident assigned to the case. This emphasis on teamwork was less true of high outliers.

Efforts to standardize resident education were also more apparent at low outliers than at high outliers. In comparison to high outliers, low outliers tended to have better-developed policies concerning the amount of direct oversight residents required generally. Several low outliers had developed very detailed criteria specifying the level and nature of attending supervision that residents must have when performing surgical procedures at each stage of their training. These criteria were usually developed through a collaborative decision-making process involving attending surgeons, attending anesthesiologists, and the nurse manager responsible for the operating room. While these criteria were not intended to override the discretionary judgment of attending surgeons, most of the surgeons with whom we spoke found the criteria helpful as a general guide. In general, high outliers were less likely to have such detailed formal policies or guidelines in place addressing the oversight of residents.

Finally, low outliers were somewhat more effective than high outliers in using peer interaction to ensure appropriate oversight of surgical residents.

While almost all of the surgical services we studied conducted meetings among attending surgeons to discuss the progress and training needs of the residents, the level of attending surgeon interaction around this issue was greater at low outliers. At one low outlier, attending surgeons met at the end of each month to discuss the progress of surgical residents and share information about how performance could be improved.

Summary
Overall, we found that in comparing low and high outliers, low outliers used a greater number and variety of coordination practices for each of the three work activities studied. As previously noted, these findings reflect general patterns and do not necessarily apply to every surgical service studied. We found examples of effective coordination practices at high outliers, albeit less frequently than we did at low outliers.

Conclusions

This chapter has reported on the relationship between objectively measured clinical outcomes and organizational practices related to coordination. The findings indicate a concurrence between the statistical model of surgical outcomes and the perceptions of experienced clinical managers and researchers. The site visits also indicated substantially different patterns of coordination between high and low outlier sites.

In investigating these relationships in detail through the survey of surgical staff, we found that coordination was more strongly related to surgical morbidity than to mortality. These results are consistent with other research and require further investigation to understand the differences in underlying processes relating to morbidity and mortality

We also found that feedback methods of coordination complement programming methods, that is, the two methods are additive. The low outliers differed from the high outliers in their greater use of both approaches to coordination.

The chapter also provides examples of specific methods of coordination. Low outlier surgical services utilized plans, rules, procedures, and protocols, not as constraints and organizational red tape, but as guidelines for routine work. In many cases, we found that effective use of standardization approaches actually allowed surgical staff greater discretion in their work. Personal approaches were useful in integrating the different professional groups involved in surgical care at both the administrative and patient care levels.

The need for health care organizations to coordinate the work of their staff is certain to increase in the future with the advent of integrated delivery systems and provider networks. In such delivery settings, patient care must be coordinated across multiple treatment levels and among health care professionals with very different clinical backgrounds and expertise. Although this study does not provide specific examples for coordinating care under these circumstances, it does indicate the important role of coordination in the process of delivering care and the potential value of combining personal and standardized coordination approaches.

Notes

The primary research comprising the content of this chapter has been reported previously (Daley et al. 1997; Young et al. 1997; Young et al. 1998).

[1] The study does have several important limitations. Two aspects of the study may limit the generalizability of the findings: the small sample size and the fact that all participants were members of one hospital system. Although a sample of 44 sites is reasonably large for an organizational study, it still imposes statistical limitations. By studying surgical services from a single hospital system, we were able to hold constant their administrative environment, systems, ownership, employment and personnel practices, and other factors. This both controlled for these factors and possibly limits generalizability of the findings.

References

Alt-White, A. C., M. Charns, and R. Strayer. 1983. Personal, organizational and managerial factors related to nurse—physician collaboration. *Nursing Administration Q* 8 (1):8-18.

Argote, L. 1982. Input Uncertainty and Organizational Coordination in Hospital Emergency Units. *Administrative Science Quarterly* 27 (3):420-434.

Baggs, J. G., S. A. Ryan, C. E. Phelps, J. F. Richeson, and J. E. Johnson. 1992. The association between interdisciplinary collaboration and patient outcomes in a medical intensive care unit. *Heart Lung* 21 (1):18-24.

Becker, S. W., S. M. Shortell, and D. Neuhauser. 1980. Management practices and hospital length of stay. *Inquiry* 17 (4):318-30.

Charns, M., and C. Lockhart. 1994. Work Design. In *Health Care Management: Organizational Design and Behavior*, edited by S. S. a. A. Kaluzny. Albany, NY: Delmar.

Charns, M. P., and M. J. Schaefer. 1983. *Health care organizations: a model for management.* Englewood Cliffs, N.J.: Prentice-Hall.

Charns, M. P., J. U. Stoelwinder, R. A. Millen, and M. J. Schaefer. 1980. Coordination and Patient Effectiveness. *Unpublished Manuscript.*

Daley, J., S. F. Khuri, W.G. Henderson, and the participants in the National VA Surgical Risk Study. 1997. Risk adjustment of the postoperative morbidity rate for the comparative assessment of the quality of surgical care: Results of the National VA Surgical Risk Study. *Journal of the American College of Surgeons* 185:328-40.

Daley, J., M. G. Forbes, G. J. Young, M. P. Charns, J. O. Gibbs, K. Hur, W. Henderson, and S. F. Khuri. 1997. Validating risk-adjusted surgical outcomes: site visit assessment of process and structure. National VA Surgical Risk Study. *Journal of the American College of Surgeons* 185 (4):341-51.

Flood, A. B. 1994. The impact of organizational and managerial factors on the quality of care in health care organizations. *Med Care Rev* 51 (4):381-428.

Georgeopoulos, B. 1986. *Organizational structure, problem solving and effectiveness.* San Francisco: Jossey-Bass.

Grover, F. L., K. E. Hammermeister, and C. Burchfiel. 1990. Initial report of the Veterans Administration Preoperative Risk Assessment Study for Cardiac Surgery. *Annals of Thoracic Surgery* 50 (1):12-26; discussion 27-8.

Grover, F. L., R. R. Johnson, G. Marshall, and K. E. Hammermeister. 1993. Factors predictive of operative mortality among coronary artery bypass subsets. *Annals of Thoracic Surgery* 56 (6):1296-306; discussion 1306-7.

Grover, F. L., R. R. Johnson, A. L. Shroyer, G. Marshall, and K. E. Hammermeister. 1994. The Veterans Affairs Continuous Improvement in Cardiac Surgery Study. *Annals of Thoracic Surgery* 58 (6):1845-51.

Haimann, T., W. G. Scott, and P. E. Connor. 1978. *Managing the modern organization.* 3d ed. Boston: Houghton Mifflin.

Hammermeister, K. E., C. Burchfiel, R. Johnson, and F. L. Grover. 1990. Identification of patients at greatest risk for developing major complications at cardiac surgery [published erratum appears in Circulation 1991 Jul;84(1):446]. *Circulation* 82 (5 Suppl):IV380-9.

Hammermeister, K. E., R. Johnson, G. Marshall, and F. L. Grover. 1994. Continuous assessment and improvement in quality of care. A model from the Department of Veterans Affairs Cardiac Surgery. *Annal of Surgery* 219 (3):281-90.

Hsiao, W. C., P. Braun, D. Yntema, and E. R. Becker. 1988a. Estimating physicians' work for a resource-based relative-value scale. *New England Journal of Medicine* 319 (13):835-41.

Hsiao, W. C., N. P. Couch, N. Causino, E. R. Becker, T. R. Ketcham, and D. K. Verrilli. 1988b. Resource-based relative values for invasive procedures performed by eight surgical specialties. *Journal of the American Medical Association* 260 (16):2418-24.

Joint Commission on Accreditation of Healthcare, Organizations. 1989. Accreditation manual for hospitals.

Kapp, M. B. 1990. 'Cookbook' medicine. A legal perspective. *Arch Intern Med* 150 (3):496-500.

Khuri, S. F., J. Daley, W. Henderson, G. Barbour, P. Lowry, G. Irvin, J. Gibbs, F. Grover, K. Hammermeister, J. F. Stremple, and et al. 1995. The National Veterans Administration Surgical Risk Study: risk adjustment for the comparative assessment of the quality of surgical care [see comments]. *Journal of the American College of Surgeons* 180 (5):519-31.

Khuri, S. F., J. Daley, W. G. Henderson, and the participants in the National VA Surgical Risk Study. 1997. Risk adjustment of the postoperative mortality rate for the comparative assessment of the quality of surgical care: Results of the National VA Surgical Risk Study. *Journal of the American College of Surgeons* 185:315-27.

Knaus, W., E. Draper, D. Wagner, and J. Zimmerman. 1987. An evaluation of outcome from intensive care in major medical centers. *Canadian Critical Care Nursing Journal* 4 (2):15.

Longest, B., and J. Klingersmith. 1994. Coordination and Communication. In *Health Care Management: Organizational Design and Behavior*, edited by S. S. a. A. Kaluzny. Albany, NY: Delmar.

March, J., and H. Simon. 1958. *Organization*. New York, NY: Wiley.

Mintzberg, H. 1979. *The Structuring of Organizations*. Englewood Cliffs, NJ: Prentice-Hall.

Mitchell, P. H., S. Armstrong, T. F. Simpson, and M. Lentz. 1989. American Association of Critical-Care Nurses Demonstration Project: profile of excellence in critical care nursing. *Heart Lung* 18 (3):219-37.

Shortell, S. M., D. M. Rousseau, R. R. Gillies, K. J. Devers, and T. L. Simons. 1991. Organizational assessment in intensive care units (ICUs): construct development, reliability, and validity of the ICU nurse-physician questionnaire. *Medical Care* 29 (8):709-26.

Shortell, S. M., J. E. Zimmerman, R. R. Gillies, J. Duffy, K. J. Devers, D. M. Rousseau, and W. A. Knaus. 1992. Continuously improving patient care: practical lessons and an assessment tool from the National ICU Study. *QRB Quality Review Bulletin* 18 (5):150-5.

Shortell, S. M., J. E. Zimmerman, D. M. Rousseau, R. R. Gillies, D. P. Wagner, E. A. Draper, W. A. Knaus, and J. Duffy. 1994. The performance of intensive care units: does good management make a difference? *Medical Care* 32 (5):508-25.

Silber, J. H., S. V. Williams, H. Krakauer, and J. S. Schwartz. 1992. Hospital and patient characteristics associated with death after surgery. A study of adverse occurrence and failure to rescue. *Medical Care* 30 (7):615-29.

Van De Ven, A. H., A .L. Delbecq, and Richard Jr Koenig. 1976. Determinants of Coordination Modes Within Organizations. *American Sociological Review* 41 (2):322-338.

Weisman, C. S., C. S. Alexander, and G. A. Chase. 1981. Determinants of hospital
    staff nurse turnover. *Medical Care* 19 (4):431-43.
Young, G. J., M. P. Charns, J. Daley, M. G. Forbes, W. Henderson, and S. F. Khuri.
    1997. Best practices for managing surgical services: the role of coordination.
    Health Care Management Review 22 (4):72-81.
Young, G. J., M. P. Charns, K. R. Desai, J. Daley, M. G. Forbes, W. Henderson, and S.
    F. Khuri. 1998. Patterns of coordination and clinical outcomes: a study of surgical
    services. *Health Services Research* 33 (5):1211-36.

Chapter 5

Implementing Continuous Quality Improvement

Robin R. Gillies, Katherine S. E. Reynolds, Stephen M. Shortell,
Edward F. X. Hughes, Peter P. Budetti, Alfred W. Rademaker,
Cheng-Fang Huang, David S. Dranove

Health care in the United States has experienced continued demands for cost reduction while maintaining quality. There is increased pressure for external accountability. One approach to deal with these challenges is the adoption of continuous quality improvement/total quality management (CQI/TQM, hereafter referred to as CQI). CQI is "an ongoing process whereby top management takes whatever steps necessary to enable everyone in the organization in the course of performing all duties to establish and achieve standards which meet or exceed the needs and expectations of their customers, both external and internal" (Miller 1996:157). Implementation of the CQI process in health care organizations has been found to be a difficult task. This chapter examines briefly the evidence regarding the extent to which CQI has been implemented in hospitals throughout the United States and uses the findings from a study of sixteen hospitals in order to identify factors that may be barriers and facilitators to the implementation of CQI.

The Status of CQI Implementation

In the past, the quality efforts in most hospitals focused on quality assurance (QA) activities, that is, a separate department, typically called the Quality Assurance Department, was charged with the detection of "after-the-fact" individual errors. However, hospitals have increasingly refocused their quality efforts on quality improvement (QI) and the principles of CQI. A number of hallmarks differentiate CQI from the QA approach. CQI is a customer-focused approach that strives to meet or exceed the needs of the customer. Customers may be internal and/or external. CQI tries to reduce variation and bring about improvement in quality or cost by eliminating system failures rather than punishing individuals. Teams of employees from multiple departments and organizational levels help identify problems and improvement opportunities in the underlying processes. The teams not only help identify problems and opportunities but are also empowered to take corrective action. Problem-solving processes are based on scientific tools, using statistical methods and measurement to identify problems and assess progress. Management is based on facts and data.

Many working in the healthcare arena view CQI as "…the strategic way of managing a *successful* hospital in the future." (McCabe 1992, emphasis added) The healthcare industry has embraced the approach, although some more reluctantly than others, "encouraged" by the Joint Commission standards that require adoption of a CQI or similar approach to improve performance. A 1993 national study (Barsness et al. 1993) showed that about 67 percent of the 3,303 responding hospitals (60 percent response rate) were using CQI methods and 48 percent had a separate CQI department. When this survey was repeated in 1998 (Arthur Andersen/American Hospital Association 1999), the percentage using CQI methods had increased to 93 percent of those responding with almost 80 percent having a separate CQI department. The hospitals are gaining more experience with the approach; in 1993, only 4 percent had used CQI methods for more than 4 years but over 41 percent had by 1998.

While the CQI approach now dominates the health care arena, evidence that its practitioners are enjoying much success (whether that be defined in terms of cost savings and/or quality) from its use is far from conclusive. Reviews of the hospital literature have found that there was little empirical research on the effectiveness of CQI, most of the supporting evidence was anecdotal, and the empirical evidence that does exist was not definitive (Bigelow and Arndt 1995; Shortell, Bennett, and Byck 1998). The 1993 and 1998 national studies, discussed above, do provide some information, at least on some of the aspects of how effective CQI efforts are in many hospitals. In these two surveys the percentage of those reporting some cost saving due to CQI efforts increased from about 40 percent to about 75 percent, although only about 7 percent in 1999 estimated that the cost savings were over $1 million. When those using CQI were asked in the two surveys to rate their satisfaction with the approach on a 1 (not satisfied at all) to 7 (very satisfied) scale, the mean level of satisfaction was 4.4 in 1993 and only 4.6 in 1998.

The CABG/THR CQI Study

The National Study for Assessing the Implementation and Impact of Clinical Quality Improvement Efforts was an effort to assess in a rigorous manner the impact of CQI, that is, whether CQI results in superior outcomes of care ascompared with other approaches to quality management. This study focused on two conditions/procedures: coronary artery bypass graft surgery (CABG) and total hip replacement (THR). There were a number of objectives of this study, hereafter referred to as the CABG/THR Study. First, the study sought to assess whether patients receiving CABG and THR in experienced CQI hospitals (in terms of both implementation of CQI and culture of the organization) do better than patients in hospitals that are much less involved or not at all involved in CQI. Hospitals that were further along in the implementation of CQI were expected to have better outcomes of care than those hospitals that were not as far along in implementation. In addition, hospitals with cultures that emphasized teamwork, cooperation, and participation were expected to have better outcomes of care than those hospitals that did not emphasize these attributes. A second objective of the study was to assess whether patients receiving care from non-CQI hospitals, but where CABG and THR caregivers have received specific CQI training, do better than patients receiving care from non-CQI hospitals where the caregivers have not been systematically exposed to such CQI training. A third objective was to examine differences in the costs of treatment for CABG and THR patients in the three study conditions — experienced CQI sites, the non-CQI sites where caregivers receive systematic education and training, and the non-CQI sites receiving no such education or training. Fourth, the study sought to measure the costs of implementing the CQI approach in the mature sites for purposes of calculating the relative cost/benefit for patients receiving care from these sites relative to the other sites. Finally, the study aimed to document the specific interventions and activities undertaken by the study hospitals to improve outcomes of care for CABG and THR.

Research Approach

Hospital Selection

Sixteen hospitals were selected to participate in the CABG/THR study. These sixteen hospitals were selected using a series of steps. First, the 5,492 hospitals listed in the 1993 AHA Guide were reduced to 760 hospitals by restricting the pool to general service, nonprofit, non-governmental, short-term care hospitals with at least 175 beds. A screening questionnaire was sent to these hospitals, asking for information regarding clinical procedures and quality efforts as well as willingness to participate in the study. Seventy-six hospitals indicated that they were willing to consider participation. Of these, forty-one were "mature" CQI hospitals and thirty-five were either "non-CQI" or "immature" CQI hospitals. Given evidence from previous studies that hospital size may play an important role in CQI implementation (O'Brien et al. 1995), the CQI and non-CQI hospitals were stratified by bed size and hospitals were randomly selected for participation in the study. Eight of the sixteen hospitals had extensive experience with CQI; four of these were 450 beds or fewer and four were larger than 450 beds. Eight hospitals had no or little experience with CQI, again with four hospitals in each bed size category. Of the eight hospitals with no or little CQI, four received training intervention (two hospitals with 450 beds or smaller and two larger than 450 beds), four did not receive training intervention.

Data Collection

Data collection was multi-faceted, attempting to gain information on the enrolled patients, the caregivers, and the hospitals. The goal was to enroll at least 200 CABG patients per hospital and at least 100 THR patients per hospital. Patient information was collected using standardized forms. Patient clinical data, including information on patient risk factors and outcomes, were collected pre-surgery, day-of-surgery, and post-surgery. In addition, the patients were surveyed regarding satisfaction at about four weeks and functional health status pre-surgery, six months post discharge, and twelve months post discharge. Patient data for the cost of each patient's hospital stay was obtained from UB92 data forms.

Culture

Data on the culture of the hospital and implementation of quality improvement was gathered via the two-part Quality Improvement Implementation Survey (QIIS) that was completed by the hospital management quality leaders as well as caregivers in CABG and THR. This instrument was distributed twice during the study (Spring/Summer 1995, n=1701; and Spring/Summer 1996, n=1744). In the first part of the QIIS, culture was assessed by asking the respondents to indicate what values, norms, and behaviors described their hospital's character, leadership, cohesion, emphases, and rewards (Quinn and Kimberly 1984; Zammuto and Krakower 1991). Based on responses to these questions, a score for each of four basic culture types was computed for each respondent. The first culture type is group culture, based on norms and values associated with affiliation, teamwork, and participation. A developmental culture is based on risk-taking innovation and change. The third type, a hierarchical culture, reflects the values and norms associated with bureaucracy. Finally, a rational culture emphasizes efficiency and achievement. Each culture type could receive a score from 0 to 100 with all four culture types adding to 100.

The scores can be conceptualized as the percent of the whole culture that is that particular culture type. No hospital, or any other organization, is likely to be totally characterized as only one of the culture types mentioned above (hierarchical score equals 100 while the scores for each of the other three culture types is 0). Hospitals are instead likely to be a combination of the culture types. In fact, this may be a necessity since hospitals, as do most other organizations, need to have at least some aspects of hierarchical (rules, stability), rational (planning, efficiency), developmental (growth), and group (participation) cultures. The crucial factor for CQI implementation is the distribution of the importance of each of these types, that is, which one(s) are predominant. Common belief is that a significant commitment to a culture emphasizing empowerment, autonomy, and risk-taking is necessary for the successful implementation of CQI. Thus, hospital cultures which emphasize group and developmental components (at least a combined score of 50) should help promote QI implementation efforts.

Implementation—Baldrige Criteria

Implementation of QI improvement was assessed based on seven scales developed from 58 items in the second part of the QIIS designed to operationalize aspects of the Malcolm Baldrige National Quality Award Criteria. The *information and analysis* scale measures to the extent to which the scope, management, and use of data and information maintain a customer focus, drive quality excellence, and improve operational and competitive performance. *Quality management* is the extent to which all work units, including research and development units and suppliers, contribute to overall quality and operational performance. *Customer satisfaction* measures the extent to which a hospital effectively orients toward customers (including patient, employee, and physician) requirements and expectations. *Quality results* are the extent to which the hospital has shown measurable improvement in quality, hospital operational performance and supplier quality. The fifth scale is *employee training*, the extent to which hospital employees are provided adequate education and training for quality improvement efforts. *Employee involvement* measures the extent to which employees are involved and empowered in the hospital's quality planning efforts. Finally, *leadership* refers to the extent to which senior executives' personal leadership and involvement creates and sustains a customer focus and clear, visible quality values and the extent to which these quality values are integrated into the hospital's management system. Scale scores for each scale were computed as the mean of the items included in the scale. The scores can range from 1, the hospital is perceived to be doing a very poor job on that dimension, to 5, the hospital is perceived as performing extremely well on that dimension, with the midpoint (3.0) on these scales indicating that the respondents perceive at best a moderate level of implementation.

Site Visits

The study also included two-day site visits conducted between December 1995 and April 1996 to eight hospitals. Four "mature" CQI, two "non-mature" CQI with no intervention, and two "non-mature" CQI with intervention were selected from the sixteen study hospitals using stratified random selection. The goal of the site visits was to learn firsthand from the hospitals participating in the study what factors facilitate or hinder quality efforts and identify "better" practices especially as they relate to CABG and THR surgery. The site visit team for each visit included three to four members, including at least one clinician. Approximately twenty-four interviews were conducted at each site. The interviews were based on written interview protocols with specific questions for top management (CEO, COO, VP Nursing), top physician leader (VP Medical Affairs or equivalent), quality leaders and members, and CABG/ THR caregiver team. Individual feedback reports were given to each hospital, and a summary report was distributed to all hospitals.

Results of the Study

One aspect of the study was the examination of the impact of a hospital's CQI maturity and culture on patient outcomes including risk adjusted mortality and morbidity, functional health status, satisfaction, and cost. Results of these empirical analyses for the CABG and THR procedures will be reported elsewhere. Although some significant relationships were found, the evidence demonstrating a CQI impact on patient outcomes was neither strong nor consistent. The focus here is on assessing the cultures and CQI implementation of the participating hospitals as well as identifying the major facilitators and barriers to quality improvement by drawing on the QIIS survey data from hospital management and caregivers and systematic observations from the site visits.

QIIS Results

Culture.

The cultures of the sixteen study hospitals were assessed using the first part of the QIIS. Given that there was very little change between the first and second administrations of the QIIS, only results from the second administration will be discussed here. The mean hospital values for each of the culture types for the second administration of the QIIS questionnaires are presented in Table 1 for the 16 study hospitals overall, the eight non-CQI hospitals, and the eight CQI hospitals. The QIIS was used in an earlier study, the Western Network Quality Improvement Study (WNQIS) (Shortell et al. 1995), and the overall study results from the 61 hospitals participating in that study are also reported in Table 1 for comparison purposes. The results for the CABG/THR Study suggest that the aspects of culture that are predominant in the sixteen hospitals in this study are the hierarchical and rational aspects with mean hospital scores of 33.2 and 28.1 respectively. On the other hand, the group and developmental culture characteristics that are conducive to CQI (such as flexibility, trust, participation and risk-taking) are much less prevalent. The group culture mean is 21.8; developmental is 17.0. The overall combined hospital mean of group and developmental is only 38.7 with a range from 29.0 to 52.0. Only one hospital had a combined group/developmental score of over 50. In comparison to the earlier WNQIS study, the sixteen CABG/THR hospitals are much less prepared culturally for CQI/TQM (Shortell et al. 1995).

Given that these overall scores combined both CQI and non-CQI hospitals, one might argue that one should not expect to see a relatively high overall group culture mean score or a relatively low hierarchical culture mean score. However, if one examines the CQI and non-CQI subsets separately, one might expect that the CQI hospitals would be characterized by much stronger group cultures and weaker hierarchical cultures than non-CQI hospitals. Looking at the mean culture values of these two sets of hospitals in Table 1, CQI hospitals do have a slightly higher group culture mean and a slightly lower hierarchical culture mean. However, none of the differences between the CQI and non-CQI hospitals is significant. For at least the sixteen hospitals involved in this study, the characteristics of the hospital cultures are not very supportive of successful CQI efforts.

	Overall Mean (n=16)	Overall Range	Non-CQI Mean (n=8)	CQI Mean (n=8)	WNQIS Mean (n=61)
Group	21.8	11.8– 32.6	20.5	23.0	32.0
Developmental	17.0	13.4– 20.7	16.5	17.4	15.6
Rational	28.1	22.4– 35.2	28.1	28.1	23.1
Hierarchical	33.2	20.8 – 37.9	34.8	31.6	28.5

Table 1. Mean Organizational Culture Scores for the Sixteen CABG/THR Hospitals

Implementation: Baldrige Criteria.

The second part of the QIIS measures perceived implementation of CQI. The mean hospital scores on the seven Baldrige scales for the second administration of the QIIS in the 16 CABG/THR Study hospitals are presented in Table 2. The scales are listed in descending order of overall mean scores. The mean hospital scores for the five equivalent scales in the WNQIS are also presented

Scale	Scale Reliability	Overall Mean (n=16)	Overall Range	Non-CQI Mean (n=8)	CQI Mean (n=8)	WNQIS Mean (N=61)
Information and analysis	0.90	3.71	3.4– 4.1	3.61	3.82*	3.70
Quality management	0.90	3.61	3.3– 3.8	3.54	3.68	3.52
Customer satisfaction	0.87	3.50	2.9– 4.1	3.38	3.62	3.67
Quality results	0.88	3.17	2.5– 3.6	3.04	3.30*	3.48
Employee training	0.79	3.15	2.6– 3.4	3.07	3.24	NA**
Employee involvement	0.87	3.15	2.5– 3.5	3.04	3.26*	NA**
Leadership	0.93	3.10	2.7– 3.6	2.99	3.24*	3.35

* Non-CQI and CQI are significantly different at p ≤0.05
**NA = No equivalent scale in WNQIS

Table 2. Mean Quality Improvement Implementation Scores for the Sixteen CABG/THR Hospitals
(1 [low] to 5 [high])

in Table 2. First, note that the overall study mean for the CABG/THR Study hospitals is below 4.0 on all of the scales. Since the range of these scales is from 1, low, to 5, high, this suggests that these hospitals are still struggling somewhat with implementing the various facets of CQI. *Information and analysis* has the highest mean score (3.71) of the seven scales. The overall mean scores for *quality management* and *customer satisfaction* are relatively high. The sixteen CABG/THR hospitals are perceived to do less well on the other scales. The overall mean scores for *quality results, employee training, employee involvement*, and *leadership* are all 3.17 or lower. Although there are minor differences in the actual values for the WNQIS hospitals, the means and the patterns are very similar for the earlier study. These results suggest that although many people in hospitals validly complain about the information systems and data problems, the greater problems may be related to training, empowerment, and leadership commitment to CQI.

Table 2 also shows the mean scores of the eight non-CQI hospitals and the eight CQI hospitals. The rankings of the various scales are the same for both sets of hospitals. The CQI hospitals mean scores are higher on all seven measures, and significantly higher on four scales. However, all scores, including those for the CQI hospitals, are still less than 4.0, indicating that these aspects of implementation are not particularly well executed in any of these hospitals.

The QIIS results from the sixteen hospitals in the CABG/THR Study regarding their culture and CQI implementation are useful in understanding why CQI may not have overwhelmed the health care arena with its success. Based on their work in the WNQIS, O'Brien et al (1995) developed a model for effective organization-wide CQI implementation. In this model, four dimensions of CQI were identified and for each dimension, the characteristics of an effective organization-wide CQI effort were suggested. The first dimension was the *cultural* dimension, that is, the beliefs, values, norms, and behaviors of the organization. The people involved must be committed to a shared purpose and to scientific principles and practices. The culture must stress teamwork, cooperation, and participation, thus allowing staff the empowerment and flexibility to make the changes that they see as necessary to improve the processes and produce continuous learning. Also important for the implementation of CQI was the *technical* dimension, referring to the techniques and tools of quality management and quality improvement. In order for an organization to be able to mount an effective CQI effort, it must be characterized by a solid foundation of technical expertise among the staff.

A third dimension crucial to CQI implementation was the *strategic* dimension. This dimension refers to the link between the organization's key strategic priorities and its CQI efforts. If CQI is to be successfully implemented in an organization, the CQI efforts and the organization's strategic plan need to be part of one another. CQI becomes the automatic way of acting and approaching problems, especially in areas of strategic priority. Roles and responsibilities are defined in terms of strategic quality goals.

The final dimension is the *structural* dimension, that is, the specific organizational structures and systems used in CQI, especially coordinating mechanisms (for example, advisory groups, steering councils, QI/QA departments, and information systems). An organization that wants to implement CQI needs to develop effective structures and systems that support the CQI effort. For example, an organization needs an effective CQI resource department and an efficient and effective steering council to keep CQI efforts on track. Given CQI emphasis on data, an organization needs a good information system that provides easily accessible data necessary to assess, improve, and evaluate. In addition, structures need to be in place to help diffuse learning throughout the organization.

Successful implementation of CQI requires that all four of these dimensions be adequately developed and aligned with each other. If any of the dimensions is not adequately developed and/or is not aligned, that is, aspects of a dimension are not "informed" by one or more of the other three dimensions, the CQI efforts will encounter problems (O'Brien et al. 1995). The results from the QIIS for the sixteen hospitals in the CABG/THR indicate that the cultural, technical, structural, and strategic dimensions are not adequately developed and/or aligned in the various study hospitals. The WNQIS results suggest that these problems are not unique to the CABG/THR Study hospitals. Underdeveloped or unaligned cultural, technical, strategic, and/or structural dimensions for many institutions appear to interfere with their CQI efforts.

Barriers to CQI Implementation

Evidence from the Site Visits
Site visits to eight of the sixteen hospitals illuminated the barriers that hinder the successful implementation of CQI and why the scores on the QIIS are not higher. The visited hospitals that seemed to be struggling with CQI

implementation were confronting a number of barriers to the development and alignment of the four dimensions mentioned above. However, it should be noted that no hospital was characterized by all of the barriers discussed below. In addition, even hospitals that seemed to be struggling had aspects of their CQI efforts that could be held up as "better practices" or positive examples that other institutions might find useful investigating.

Environment

Before discussing the barriers directly related to the cultural, technical, strategic, and structural dimensions, however, several more general "environmental" barriers should be mentioned. One factor preventing the building of the foundations of CQI is the lack of managed care activity in the hospital's geographic area. This reduces concern, especially among physicians, for developing the most *efficient* quality care. In addition, at the time of the site visits the lack of external organizations requesting quality data in order to make purchasing or credentialling decisions meant that most hospitals felt less pressure to develop the skills and tools necessary to provide such data.

Cultural Dimension

As seen in the results of the culture survey, the values and norms of most of the hospitals in the current study are not based on affiliation, teamwork, and participation. Evidence from the site visits suggests this lack of "group" orientation continues for a number of reasons. At many of the hospitals, recognition and awards are given to individuals. Performance appraisals emphasize individual activity rather than team activity and the good of the larger community (the service or hospital). Organizational and psychological barriers exist among departments limiting the extent to which people are willing to participate in cross-unit projects and, even more importantly, make decisions based on the collective good rather than their own departments. In many cases, projects are characterized by a lack of follow-through after an initial big effort to start the project. Most of the hospitals visited lacked physician "champions;" in some cases none exist and in other cases only a few, overburdened ones exist. Because of the lack of physician commitment, many hospitals are unwilling to make changes (for example, modify clinical practices, redesign the structure, require involvement) that physicians may find unacceptable. The hospital administrators are concerned that changes may cause physicians to refer their patients to other hospitals.

Technical Dimension

Technical barriers also exist. Most of the hospitals have provided CQI training to at least some of the relevant personnel. Typically, however, physicians are the last group of those affiliated with the hospital to receive training, and there continues to be a lack of widespread physician involvement in the QI process. The results from the 1993 and 1998 national QI surveys (Barsness et al. 1993; Arthur Andersen/American Hospital Association 1999) reinforce these site visit observations from the CABG/THR Study. These surveys reported that the average percentage of personnel trained in CQI was about 22 percent in 1993 and about 35 percent in 1998. Only about 11 percent of personnel had participated on QI teams in 1993 increasing to about 21 percent four years later. However, even by 1998 only about 22 percent of the physicians had been trained in CQI and about the same percentage participated on QI teams. This lack of physician involvement is perhaps the most common and troublesome barrier that CQI efforts encounter.

Another technical barrier is that some of those who have received basic CQI training have not been able to put their new training to use. Consequently, many fail to retain the skills. CQI support personnel often are not available to help guide and provide data, thus, often stalling projects. Clinical or managerial personnel must often perform support tasks such as clerical work that misdirects their talents. In a number of cases, those involved in the CQI efforts lacked an understanding of what the actual clinical practices and processes were, and were thus unable to assess problems and design solutions.

Strategic Dimension

Many of the hospitals also confront a number of strategic barriers. One of the major strategic barriers is that there is often no linkage between a hospital's (and its units') quality improvement plans and strategic business plans. These plans often operate independently of one another. Therefore, CQI efforts often have little or no strategic importance. Second, many organizations are unable to identify levers of change to produce desired strategic outcomes.

Structural Dimension
Many hospitals also confront a number of structural barriers. For example, larger hospitals find that their size inhibits effective interaction and communication. Some hospitals had too many committees involved in the approval process of quality improvement. Often, hospital commitment of resources to CQI activities (for example, CQI department, clerical support, paid time for participation) is inadequate. At many of the visited hospitals, parts of a clinical service line functioned independently of the rest of the service line. For example, it was very common for the cardiovascular operating room team to function with very little communication with the rest of the cardiovascular team. At all of the sites visited, the information systems were deemed by those interviewed to be inadequate. The existing information systems were designed to produce QA data rather than data that are more useful to QI efforts. Most interviewees also felt that insufficient funds were being dedicated to the development of the hospital information system. Some hospitals had multiple data departments, each of which often guarded "its" data very closely and was reluctant to cooperate with other data departments or give information to individual clinical units. Information systems (as well as personal computers) often were unable to "talk to each other."

Facilitators of CQI Implementation — The Case of Hospital A
The barriers discussed above characterize to one degree or another, the CQI efforts of most of the hospitals in the study that received site visits. However, the site visits also reveal a number of positive examples of CQI implementation. Details of the experience of one of the hospitals that received a site visit, which will be called *Hospital A*, help illuminate the factors that facilitate the implementation of CQI.

Environment
The market environment for Hospital A at the time of the visit was predominantly fee-for-service, but hospital leadership felt that managed care in some form would be impacting on the area and would necessitate greater focus on quality improvement and reporting. The hospital had reorganized from a traditional function-based hospital with all the requisite departments to a focus on centers, including the business center, the care centers (cardiac,

medical/surgery, family, surgery, and outpatient), and the support center. Cutting across the care centers were service lines, each with a service line leader (called an "investigator"). Although Hospital A reorganized and restructured, any downsizing was accomplished primarily through attrition, not through layoffs. The hospital had been characterized by a great deal of continuity in its leadership and staff—many of whom had been with the hospital for many years, advancing in the organization over time. The leadership team was relatively small; the hospital did not have a number of the traditional vice-presidents (such as Human Resources and Strategy). These functions were handled in the care centers.

Cultural Dimension
Hospital A's culture was described as very open, employee-centered and customer-focused. Communication seemed to be very good. The culture appeared to be a one that is conducive to learning. In addition, the culture encouraged risk taking and was not seen as punishment oriented. A major orientation of Hospital A's culture was to apply CQI principles. The hospital was very team oriented and had a number of self-directed, multi-disciplinary teams. There were no "Employee of the Year" awards, only recognition of team efforts. This team-orientation was further reinforced by the hospital's policy of "gain-sharing," in which rewards were distributed only if all segments of the hospital met their goals. Gain-sharing helped many see the larger picture; for example, personnel found floating to other units less objectionable because they understood how this helped the functioning of the hospital. Many employees felt empowered and saw the hospital as a self-governing institution. Improvement was a central concept. The attitude of many employees was that they can do everything better. However, they understood that they needed to prioritize their efforts. Customer satisfaction was highly valued by most employees, an attitude that was reinforced by hospital policy to include customer satisfaction measures in its performance appraisals.

Hospital leadership seemed widely respected and was considered to have a great deal of integrity. The hospital management culture appeared innovative in nature. There was generally strong board support for the quality efforts including a committee on performance. This was aided by the fact that some of the board members were familiar with quality improvement from a non-health care perspective.

Strategic Dimension

Hospital A was also very strong on the strategic dimension. Quality was an important part of the hospital's philosophy. The hospital did not have a strategic "business" plan, but rather a strategic "quality" plan. CQI was a key part of the hospital's strategic quality plan and was actually written into the plan. In addition, very importantly, there was widespread knowledge of the hospital's strategic quality plan among the hospital community.

The key to Hospital A's approach was their *alignment and deployment process* whereby the quality improvement and performance initiatives in each of the hospital's major care centers were directly linked to the hospital's overall mission and strategic goals. These care centers developed their own improvement objectives within their areas. Any quality improvement activity that an individual or unit wanted to undertake had to be a part of each care center's alignment and deployment plan which was itself directly linked to the hospital's strategic quality plan. The strategic alignment and deployment process included a 90-day accountability process whereby each executive and care team leader translated overall goals and objectives into a 90-day period for accomplishment, and were then reviewed based on that accomplishment at the end of 90 days. The process also included rating potential CQI projects according to criteria related to strategic quality plan and pursuing those with the highest score.

Technical Dimension

This hospital was also very strong on the technical dimension. First, almost every employee at Hospital A received quality improvement training over the years. Moreover, many of those employed by the hospital had received or were scheduled to receive more advanced training. Hospital A commonly benchmarked itself against other organizations throughout the country. In order to monitor the performance of the hospital and its components, it developed a set of dashboard measures. Similar to a driver being able to monitor the functioning of an automobile using the dashboard instruments, those responsible for hospital performance used selected indicators to monitor its functioning in terms of its strategic quality plan's goals and objectives. The extensive use of control and run charts for long periods of time enabled the hospital to monitor continuously, so that improvements were sustainable. The hospital was working to refine its dashboard measures and reduced them to four key areas: market position, customer satisfaction, cost/price leadership and clinical outcomes. Each care center had its own dashboard measures, but these were linked to the hospital's dashboard measures. Good use was made of graphic data based primarily on control and run charts using longitudinal data over time. The expectation was that presentations would be based on data and these tools, and if this format was not followed, reports were not well received.

Structural Dimension
The hospital also had some structural factors that facilitated CQI. A number of mechanisms were in place for transferring best practices. These included a care center leadership group, a team leadership group, and a quality council. The care centers allowed the hospital to develop more of a cross-functional approach to patient care that cuts across departments. This incorporated the best principles of patient focused care without massive structural changes in building design. Each care center had a facilitator, that is, someone who helped provide resources so others could do what was needed to done. The hospital developed a strong quality resource group of 6 to 7 people that provided impetus and help for quality efforts. This resource group appeared to be especially adept at persuading and cajoling the physicians to forge ahead with their quality improvement efforts. The members of the group understood the importance of having good data when working with physicians. Strong middle management linked the organization's strategic quality plan with day-to-day activities. The redesign of the hospital structure from one of departments to one of care centers across functional teams helped removed some of the old communication barriers. Nurse manager meetings and care center leader meetings that cut across the divisions within the hospital also aided communication.

Continuing Barriers to Implementation
This is not to say that Hospital A had not experienced any problems. As was the case in all the other hospitals visited, one of the major problems Hospital A faced was the rather marked lack of physician involvement in the hospital's quality improvement efforts. There appeared to be a relative lack of physician leadership for total quality management work. No physician "champions" existed to help get the other physicians on board. Most of the physicians appeared to be only tangentially involved to the hospital's quality improvement efforts. The fee-for-service environment did not provide any incentive for the

extra burden of participation in quality improvement work, especially given that most the physicians were extremely busy in their practices. In addition, many physicians were suspicious of the data collected for CQI, concerned that it would be used to punish them. The lack of physician involvement sometimes meant that some quality improvement projects were not undertaken for fear that they may offend the doctors. This lack of involvement of a substantial segment of the hospital community limits the degree to which CQI can be successful. The lack of involvement is especially critical for physicians because most observers who discuss the potential for CQI indicate that it will be successful in the clinical arena only if physicians "buy-in" to the approach.

The hospital also encountered other barriers. Some described the culture as still in transition. The hospital leadership was very much oriented towards preparing the hospital to compete in a managed care environment. However, the board and many physicians were more oriented toward the current fee-for-service world. Most of the hospital staff seemed to believe that the future will be one of managed care and increased competition; there were, however, a "handful of change resistors." Like most hospitals, Hospital A's information systems were not adequate — they did not easily provide the required data nor link financial and clinical data. Although CQI training had been widespread, the CQI approach had not become so ingrained that it is automatic way to approach problems. In particular, more systemic thinking needed to occur at the middle management and lower levels in the organization. As at many other hospitals, the same people were repeatedly involved in CQI efforts, and some seemed to be close to "burning out." It was sometimes difficult to get the right people together and to develop ownership of a project. The lack of resources, especially time (even though most quality work was done on paid time), inhibited efforts. Lack of training for staff in new positions of responsibility hindered their ability to take on the new roles with confidence and increased skepticism towards cross-training.

Status of Implementation
Hospital A had one of the strongest CQI programs, at least in terms of implementation of the approach of the hospitals visited. Whether this evaluation would stand if all sixteen hospitals had been visited is obviously unknown, but evidence from the QIIS culture and implementation survey support the conclusion that this hospital should have a comparatively strong CQI program.

Hospital A had the highest score for group culture (32.1), the lowest on hierarchical culture (20.8), and the only combined group/developmental culture score over 50 (52.0). It scored the highest of all of the hospitals on five of the seven Baldrige implementation scales, including scores of about 4.0 on the customer satisfaction scale and the information and analysis scale. On the remaining two scales, employee quality training and employee quality planning involvement, it was second highest. However, these results indicate that many at the hospital perceived much work still needs to be done. In fact, Hospital A's quality efforts reflect its barriers and facilitators—it has had some successes but continues to face challenges.

Other Facilitators
While the example of Hospital A illustrates many practices that facilitate CQI implementation, additional examples from other hospitals visited should be noted. At one of the hospitals, physicians were compensated and acknowledged for their QI activities. This helped increase physician participation. Management at one hospital sought input from physicians and clinical teams in formulating the hospital's strategic business plan. One hospital instituted a CQI carnival to demonstrate that learning can be fun as well as to communicate the various CQI activities to the staff. The carnival was taped so that an edited tape could be used to kick off a second round of CQI employee training. In addition, a live scaled-down version of the carnival was also taken to affiliated nursing home. At several hospitals, patients were used as a resource for the development of the education packet, including a critical pathway for patient and family that presented in layperson terms, expectations for recovery.

Conclusions

Many other examples of ways to help develop or align aspects of the four dimension of CQI implementation could be related from not only the CABG/THR Study but also from the vast array of journals, newsletters, and conference which seek to share the experiences of those trying to develop CQI programs. However, at this point, for the sixteen hospitals in the CABG/THR study as well as many of the hospitals throughout the United States, the barriers to implementation are greater than the facilitators. Perhaps Arndt and Bigelow

(1995) are correct when they suggest that CQI may not be suited to the health care environment and may never be successful regardless of how long it is employed? However, implementation and use of CQI does not occur in a vacuum. The customer focus and empowerment aspects of CQI require that organizations have certain attributes to ensure effective implementation. The cultural, technical, strategic, and structural dimensions must be developed and aligned in order to give CQI a chance to be successful. At this point few, if any, hospitals have sufficiently developed these four dimensions to allow the full implementation of CQI.

Evaluations of CQI's effectiveness are, at this point, incomplete, and it would be inappropriate to make decisions about its merits in the health sector, given the state of the information. What is most appropriate now is for each organization using CQI, to evaluate its implementation of the approach, identify its own barriers and facilitators, and focus on the full implementation of CQI. A number of researchers or practitioners in healthcare discuss implementation (see Griffith, Sahney, and Mohr 1995; Gaucher and Coffey 1993; Kaluzny, McLaughlin, and Kibbe 1992; McLaughlin and Kaluzny 1990; McLaughlin 1995). Key to these and other discussions is the paramount importance of leadership, commitment and patience and the involvement of physicians in the process. It is also crucial that governing boards understand the need for CQI. CQI efforts need to extend across the complete continuum of care, both inpatient and outpatient. The process of implementing CQI is not easy. Only a fully implemented CQI approach will permit the kind of evaluation that will truly test its value in health care.

Notes

This research was supported by the Agency for Health Care Policy and Research (Grant #RO1 HS08523), the Baxter-Allegiance Foundation, Bristol-Myers Squibb, the Center for Health Management Research of The Network for Healthcare Management Education, and the National Science Foundation. Appreciation is expressed to the National Advisory Committee members, Paul Batalden, M.D., Donald Berwick, M.D., David Gustafson, Ph.D., Brent James, M.D., Phil Nudelman, D. Pharm., James Roberts, M.D., and Vin Sahney, Ph.D., for their advice and support, Albert L. Siu, M.D. for his comments on an earlier draft, and Matthew H. Liang, M.D. and Steven Stern, M.D. for their assistance. Recognition is also due those who provided research assistance throughout the study: Algernon Austin, Marjorie Duncan, Shahnaz Hussain, Angela Johnson, Michaela Kotrckova, Elizabeth Lock, Nina Nohejlova, Elizabeth Reite, Juliana Shortell, Tasha Shoup, Melissa Solomon, Amy Steckel, Cynthia Tenny, and Corinne Wildenradt.

Participating hospitals were: Alta Bates Medical Center, Berkeley, CA; Bellin Hospital, Green Bay, WI; Carondelet St. Mary's/St. Joseph's Hospitals, Tucson, AZ; St. Joseph Mercy Hospital, Ann Arbor, MI; Cedars-Sinai Medical Center, Los Angeles, CA; Charleston Area Medical Center, Charleston, WV; Christ Hospital and Medical Center, Oak Lawn, IL; Cooper Hospital/University Medical Center, Camden, NJ; Grant/ Riverside Methodist Hospitals, Columbus, OH; Lutheran General Hospital, Park Ridge, IL; Meriter Hospital, Madison, WI; Mills-Peninsula Hospitals, Burlingame, CA; Presbyterian Hospital (Presbyterian Healthcare Services), Albuquerque, NM; Providence Medical Center, Seattle, WA; Sherman Hospital, Elgin, IL; and St. Luke's Hospital, Cedar Rapids, IA.

References

Arthur Andersen/American Hospital Association. 1999. *The National Hospital Quality Improvement Survey*. Knowledge Leadership Series, Issue 3. Chicago, IL.

Arndt, M., and B. Bigelow. 1995. The Implementation of Total Quality Management in Hospitals: How Good is the Fit? *Health Care Management Review* 20(5):7-14.

Barsness, Z. I., S. M. Shortell, R. R. Gillies, E. F. X. Hughes, J. L. O'Brien, D. Bohr, C. Izui, and P. Kralovec. 1993. The Quality March. *Hospital & Health Networks* 5:52-6.

Bigelow, B., and M. Arndt. 1995. Total Quality Management: Field of Dreams? *Health Care Management Review* 20 (5):15-25.

Gaucher, E. J., and R. J. Coffey.1993. *Total Quality in Healthcare: From Theory to Practice*. San Francisco: Jossey-Bass.

Griffith, J. R., V. K. Sahney, and R. A.. Mohr. 1995. *Reengineering Health Care: Building on CQI*. Ann Arbor, MI: Health Administration Press.

Kaluzny, A.D., C.P. McLaughlin, and D.C. Kibbe (1992) "Continuous Quality Improvement in the Clinical Setting: Enhancing Adoption," *Quality Management in Health Care*, 1:37-44.

McCabe, W.J. 1992. Total Quality Management in a Hospital. *Quality Review Bulletin*, April. 134-40.

McLaughlin, C.P., and A.D. Kaluzny. 1990. Total Quality Management in Health: Making it Work. *Health Care Management Review* 15 (1):7-14.

McLaughlin, C.P. 1995. Quality Management in Health Care: Success and Lessons in Implementation. *Journal of Continuing Education in the Health Professions* 15 (3):165-74.

Miller, W. J. 1996. A Working Definition for Total Quality Management (TQM) Researchers. *Journal of Quality Management* I.2:149-59.

O'Brien, J. L., S. M. Shortell, E. F. X. Hughes, R. W. Foster, J. M. Carman, H. Boerstler, and E. J. O'Connor. 1995. An Integrative Model for Organization-wide Quality Improvement: Lessons from the Field. *Quality Management in Health Care* 3(4): 19-30.

Quinn, R. E., and J. R. Kimberly. 1984. Paradox, Planning, and Perseverance: Guidelines for Managerial Practice. In *Managing Organization Transitions*, edited by J. R. Kimberly and R. E. Quinn. Homewood, IL: Dow Jones-Irwin.

Shortell, S. M., J. L. O'Brien, J. M. Carman, R. W. Foster, E. F. X. Hughes, H. Boerstler, and E. J. O'Connor. 1995. Assessing the Impact of Continuous Quality Improvement/Total Quality Management: Concept versus Implementation. *Health Services Research*,30 (2):377-401.

Shortell, S. M., C. L. Bennett, G. R. Byck. 1998. Assessing the Impact of Continuous Quality Improvement on Clinical Practice: What Will It Take to Accelerate Progress? *The Milbank Quarterly* 76(4):593-624.

Zammuto, R. F., and J. Y. Krakower. 1991. Quantitative and Qualitative Studies of Organizational Culture. *Organizational Change and Development* 5:83-114.

Chapter 6

Evaluation Units in French Hospitals: Experiences and Limitations

Isabelle Durand-Zaleski and Pierre Durieux

Health sector quality and its measurement emerged as an important issue in France from the mid-1980's. Successive governments have passed regulations to ensure that health care providers are accountable for the quality of care and a 1991 hospital law mandated that "health care facilities should develop policies to evaluate professional practices, organization of care and any action contributing to patient care so as to guarantee its quality and efficiency". The so-called "Juppé reform", promulgated in 1996, introduced mandatory accreditation procedures for all hospitals (Colin and Geffroy 1997). At the same time, cost-containment strategies and hospital cost control using a global budgeting process were implemented. Hospitals were also required to use clinical guidelines similar to those developed in the private sector (*références médicales*)[1] and began to face the challenges of quality and costs.

This chapter discusses an important result of health sector transition in France, the development of Evaluation Units (EUs) and the role of quality in their activities. We also examine broader issues related to quality assurance and accreditation in the French health sector.

The Current Situation

The French healthcare system is currently undergoing major reform, initiated by Parliament in April 1996. The major goal of this reform was to modify the financing system for health care. Regional authorities are in charge of management and strategic planning for all hospitals in a given area. Regional authorities also have to ensure equal access to care and quality of care in hospitals under their jurisdiction. They have budgetary powers, can restructure the supply of hospital care within a region and can use quality of care as a criterion when allocating hospital budgets.

Another important aspect of the reform legislation is the mandatory recording of computerized information, both by hospitals (using a DRG system) and by physicians in private practice. With regard to patient satisfaction, the 1996 laws mandate that hospitals produce and enforce a charter of patient rights and administer discharge questionnaires to assess patient satisfaction. The legislation also created a national Agency, ANAES (*Agence nationale d'accréditation et d'évaluation en santé*)[2], responsible for the accreditation of health care institutions and the promotion of medical practice evaluation. The accreditation procedures, being proposed and introduced on a pilot basis in France, are expected to be similar to those in other countries (Shaw and Brooks 1991) and involve self-evaluation and site-visits by external quality auditors. It is likely that the results of the accreditation procedures will be publicly available to permit comparisons between institutions, although it will not be possible to compare specific medical departments within and between hospitals.

Prior to the development of accreditation, the French Social Security system, which is responsible for the largest proportion of provider reimbursement, had not initiated or promoted quality assurance programs. Consequently, quality in health care was mainly left in the hands of medical associations, researchers and public health professionals. Interest in health care quality assurance in France began to grow in the early 1990s, when some researchers considered adapting industrial quality assurance approaches to the hospital setting. Several hospitals in the AP-HP group, the regional public hospital system for the Paris metropolitan area[3], served as pilot sites for such projects (de Pouvourville 1997). For example, Hôpital Louis Mourier developed a pilot project to improve drug dispensing (Fontaine et al. 1993) and several other projects were implemented including improving operating room management, emergency departments, prevention of hospital-acquired infections and the quality of medical records.

In 1994, the PAQ (*Programme assurance qualité*), a special fund to finance quality assurance programs in hospitals was created by the Ministry of Health with the support of ANDEM. More than 50 hospitals got such funding, but the program stopped in 1997 and, as it has not been evaluated, its impact is unclear.

Evaluation Units in French Hospitals

Whilst formal quality assurance initiatives may be a recent phenomenon, Evaluation Units (EUs) have existed in French hospitals since the end of the 1970s. EUs are responsible for medical evaluation, including the development of practice guidelines and share with the hospital's administration, the responsibility for accreditation and the implementation of quality assurance programs. They were first established in individual hospitals and hospital groups such as AP-HP (Fontaine et al. 1997). Currently, more hospitals have established EUs and nearly every university hospital in France has one, either operating independently or shared with another institution. The driving force behind the increasing number of EUs is believed to be the legal requirement for the implementation of evaluation procedures in hospitals. However, the scope of activity of EUs has widened to include assistance in the design of clinical trials, cost-containment programs and teaching.

A recent survey of Public Health departments and EUs in 17 hospitals in the Paris region revealed substantial differences in structure and staffing. EUs were independent departments in about half the hospitals studied and about a quarter had a research affiliation. They are generally run by public health physicians, half of whom are oriented towards biostatistics and medical informatics, the remainder being specialized in medical economics and epidemiology. About one-third had physicians with interests in all the aforementioned areas. The average number of physicians per unit was approximately 3.5 with additional staff comprising a technician and a secretary.

EUs tasks within hospitals included management of the medical information system, participation in evaluation and quality assurance and, more recently, preparation for the accreditation process. Physicians working in EUs were often active members of hospital committees in areas such as drug policy, hospital-acquired infections, finance, clinical research, medical informatics and evaluation. EUs performed roughly two-thirds of their clinical research within their own hospital, the remainder for hospitals that do not possess such units or for industry. On average, EUs participated in 10 research projects, about a third of which were multi-center trials.

With regard to organizational issues, the survey showed that most heads of EUs wished their unit to operate as an independent department, loosely associated with other hospital structures involved in quality assurance, and separate from the hospital administration. The chairpersons of hospital medical boards viewed the EUs as very likely to be effective advocates for quality improvement in hospitals because of their close interaction with the clinical departments, the medical management of the hospital, and also with the general headquarters of the Paris hospitals consortium. Hospital directors saw the strength of EUs as their expertise in the application of evaluation and quality assurance methods and their major weakness as their lack of visibility within the hospital and the paucity of information about the services that they provided. Management wished to merge EUs and information technology (IT) with administrative services, on the grounds that all were involved in managing the hospital information systems, quality assurance programs and accreditation processes. Further tasks of EUs, according to hospital directors and medical managers, were the management of the hospital archives and intranet.

Evaluation Units: The Assistance Publique-Hopitaux de Paris Experience

Medical Evaluation

Medical evaluation, as practiced by hospital EUs, is defined as the study of patient management to detect variations from an agreed norm and the design of corrective measures. Among such measures is the implementation of clinical guidelines. Medical evaluation, as understood in French hospitals, differs from quality assurance because it is only concerned with the medical component of the process of care, and thus has a close relationship with academic research and public health.

The tools available to EUs include those provided by the hospital clinical and administrative information system such as diagnostic and procedure codes and length of stay data. In addition, information systems often exist in technical departments and the hospital pharmacy, although it may be impossible to link these to the main database. Other data sources include the hospital accounting and financial system, although these systems do not currently collect data on individual patients.

Thus, ad-hoc evaluation often requires that evaluation physicians design prospective studies, with the assistance of clinicians and nurses. This provides an opportunity to explain and spread the culture of evaluation within the hospital. The most important targets for evaluation are sentinel events, distinguished by their frequency, severity or associated expense. Economic analysis is also becoming a feature of evaluation, although the current financing system of French university hospitals limits their usefulness (Durieux and Ravaud 1997).

Most hospitals have developed their own evaluation tools with a special focus, at least as far as the AP-HP group is concerned, on the evaluation of medical procedures, diagnostic test and drug prescribing, pain management, terminal care, quality of medical records and hospital-acquired infections. The evaluation philosophy is that quality defects are the result of faulty organization and not faulty behavior (Donabedian 1989). Medical evaluation follows the traditional steps of literature review, design, validation and the implementation of practice guidelines. Modification of the request or order form for tests or for drugs is an important quality improvement intervention (Henderson 1982; Zaat, Eijk and Bonte 1992). Other guidelines, such as the Ottawa Ankle Rules, have been implemented via education, feedback and the use of reminders (Audelely et al. 1997).

A study of the Ottawa Ankle Rules demonstrated the relevance of a prediction rule developed in Canada, to health care organizations in France. A limited strategy (posters mounted in the emergency department) resulted in a persistent improvement in the management of ankle injuries. Practice guidelines or clinical rules are now widely used and it is important to demonstrate that they improve the quality of care (Weingarten 1997). Guidelines should be subjected to rigorous evaluation, as would be required for any new drug or technology and we consider that EUs, particularly in the university hospital setting, can play a pivotal role in these evaluations.

The choice of guidelines for evaluation depends on the hospital's priorities and is often determined by the possible savings that could result from their implementation. It has been difficult, thus far, to implement identical guidelines in all AP-HP hospitals, let alone at a national level. The reasons for the reluctance to standardize practice guidelines may be related to differences in hospital case-mix, which can influence the predictive value and therefore the relevance of tests, and the likelihood of therapeutic success or failure (Durand-Zaleski et al. 1993). Other reasons include conflicts of interests, where a reduction in the number of tests prescribed would result in fewer resources being allocated to a certain department, controversy concerning the medical evidence in support of a certain protocol, and the absence of committed leadership.

It is important to consider the standardization of not only the request forms but also of report forms, to ensure quality of care. In a prospective study, we assessed clinician agreement in the interpretation of lung scan reports to diagnose pulmonary embolism and found that physicians reading the same narrative routine diagnostic report reached different conclusions. This finding was used in the implementation of standardized nuclear medicine reports (Bastuji-Garin, Schaeffer, and Wolkenstein et al. 1998).

Management Audit at Créteil Hospital

In 1994, Créteil hospital, a member of the AP-HP group, initiated a systematic audit of every medical and technical department. The audit aimed to improve the organization of individual departments, the allocation of resources and the quality of patient management. The audits were supervised by the medical management of the hospital, and performed by doctors, nurses and administrators from Créteil hospital and other French and foreign hospitals. The audit was motivated by the legislative reform of hospital operations (Loi Hospitalière, July 24 1987 and July 31 1991). These laws, and similar regulations, mandated that an "audit and reform procedure" be performed by every public hospital department chairman every fifth year. The nature of this procedure was not clearly specified by law, and was thus decided upon by the hospital medical staff and management. Créteil hospital decided to seize this opportunity and organize a management audit of each department every fifth year. The objective of the audit was to identify strengths and weaknesses, areas for improvement, and to suggest follow-up indicators, both quantitative and qualitative (Derry and Lawrence 1991). A survey committee was created for each department audited, to collect data, analyze results and present recommendations. The members were chosen according to the medical specialty being audited and included physicians, surgeons, a representative of the faculty, a representative of the non-medical personnel, a public health specialist, the hospital director and the president of the medical board. After auditing a department, a process that included interviews with personnel inside and outside the department, the committee produced explicit recommendations for the next five years. These recommendations were then presented to the department's chief, who validated both the report and the evaluation criteria proposed. Quantitative criteria to assess compliance with the recommendations after five years have only recently been introduced.

Audit has proven to be a useful problem-solving tool. The participation of foreign experts has facilitated strategic development and the anticipation of problems that have been identified in other countries. The audit process, in our experience, has sources of inefficiency similar to those found in industry. It is hampered by the lack of a proper information system, a crisis in the department, ambiguous departmental objectives, the lack of personnel buy-in, and an environment (academic or financial constraints) which limits the possibilities for change. The results of one such audit, performed in the Créteil Hospital radiology department, have been published, permitting critical academic comment on the procedure (Durand-Zaleski et al. 1996).

Resource Allocation

Allocating resources among departments is a common problem for hospital managers. Although part of the allocation is self-decided under a prospective payment system, hospital departments present competing programs for the remaining funding. These programs often involve new technologies. Hospital resources are claimed by departments (clinical or laboratory) that wish to acquire a new diagnostic or therapeutic apparatus, or introduce a currently available procedure.

The Evaluation Unit at Créteil Hospital was asked to develop a procedure for prioritizing the proposed acquisition programs. A committee was created to design an evaluation tool and implement a rating method, collect and analyze results and present recommendations to the medical management and hospital director. This committee had 8 members, 7 of whom were doctors and one an administrator. The evaluation tool was designed to assess four dimensions: improvement in the quality of patient care, feasibility, value for teaching and research, and compatibility with the hospital's strategic goals. Each dimension was assessed with a questionnaire containing 4 to 11 items. The relative weights given to each dimension reflected the priorities of the hospital. We used a linear model approach, summing the scores of the individual items in each dimension. Acceptance of differences between the amounts allocated to each department was facilitated by transparency and general knowledge of financing across programs. Clinical departments tended to have higher scores than technical departments, which led to the separation of financing procedures. The final score of a program was regarded as only one element in the discussion, the other elements including total cost of the program, as well as more "political" considerations (Durand-Zaleski et al. 1994).

The Development of Quality Assurance and Accreditation Programs

There is currently an initiative underway to have all AP-HP hospitals reach agreement on uniform evaluation criteria within and between hospitals. These criteria could also be used for budgeting purposes. Accreditation and quality assurance are major components of current French health care reform. As in other countries, the objectives include continuous quality improvement and improved patient satisfaction. In French hospitals where EUs have been created, their missions may encompass a large range of tasks, the relative importance of which depend on local factors and priorities. Some hospitals have initiated their own quality assurance procedures, often with the help of consulting firms. They have often used existing safety and certification laws and regulations. France, like most industrialized countries, has legislation defining the equipment and staffing of operating theaters, intensive care units, and emergency departments. In addition to medical regulations, other legal requirements concern fire safety, food, waste disposal and aspects of running a large enterprise. Technical departments such as radiology, pathology, virology and nuclear medicine in various hospitals across the country have initiated an ISO certification process. The choice between waiting for accreditation or seeking ISO certification has so far been made without any legal or institutional mandate. Hospital departments that perform technical tasks are candidates for ISO certification, unlike wards or clinical departments that perform medical or nursing procedures, and are thus more likely to rely on accreditation. When preparing for ISO certification, departments have seldom required assistance from EUs, except to initiate the procedures and provide explanations on the different methods of quality assurance. Some hospitals obtained certification of some of their activities (ISO norms). However, due to the development of accreditation, it is unclear as to whether or not the ISO certification procedure will persist in the French health sector.

The role of the EUs in the accreditation process is currently being discussed and will include involvement in the early phase of self evaluation and the provision of methodological support for clinical departments, imaging departments and laboratories. Non-clinical issues such as logistics and administration will be dealt with by administrators. There is currently no plan for academic accreditation of resident training in either clinical departments or laboratories.

Legislation was enacted between 1982 and 1995 dealing with risk management, the reporting of adverse drug effects and problems related to the use of human tissues and cells, organs, blood, and other medical material. Reporting is mandatory and is organized by individual hospitals, with a responsible physician, usually assisted by a committee. Evaluation physicians participate in this committee and give methodological advice.

Future Challenges

There is growing pressure from the French government, health policy makers, health insurers and the public to improve quality of health care institutions. Since 1991, several laws have required the implementation of quality interventions and a mandatory accreditation procedure will soon exist for health care institutions. An increasing number of hospitals have established EUs to develop quality and evaluate medical care. Quality initiatives are also underway at a regional level. These initiatives, developed by a variety of groups, include medical and nursing audit, implementation of clinical guidelines, quality assurance and, more recently, total quality management. EUs are also sometimes involved in others projects such as the management of information systems, risk management, prevention of hospital-acquired infection, the organization of care and resource allocation.

Most physicians now accept EUs, as they are aware of the current scientific and economic context of medical practice and their responsibilities. Physicians are beginning to accept some scrutiny and control of their practices, despite the fact that current concepts of evidence-based medicine and health economics were not part of their medical school training.

Certain barriers to the implementation of quality management initiatives however, remain. Hospitals are generally poorly organized and hospital physicians have a high level of autonomy since they are appointed by the state (the Ministry of Health or the University), and not by the hospital. They are thus relatively independent of the hospital administration, and as hospital physicians are generally highly specialized, they often do not consider organizational problems as important.

We have already stressed that hospital information systems are often poor. These systems are built to assist in the general administration of the hospital and are not designed to evaluate the quality of care. Consequently, evaluation has mostly focused on the process of care, with only limited attention to outcomes. Events such as the blood transfusion scandal raised doubts about the quality of activities of some health professionals and institutions. Many health professionals and the public worry that efforts to reduce the cost of health care services will decrease quality of care. The simultaneous development of quality assurance programs and cost-containment strategies has generated some skepticism amongst health providers. There are advantages and disadvantages in incorporating EUs into the hospital administration. In our view, EUs and hospital administrators do not necessarily have similar goals when it comes to the evaluation of practices. Due to financial constraints, the annual budgeting process, and the short term nature of hospital budgeting horizons (3 years on average), hospital directors may be tempted to favor immediate action over long term policies. Evaluation doctors operating from a public health viewpoint may have a different perspective on what constitutes the best interests of the hospital. There are obvious areas of interaction between the hospital management and EUs in particular with regard to accreditation, quality assurance and medical information systems and EUs have a vital role in driving quality improvement in the French health sector.

Notes

[1] These guidelines are, however, not mandatory; unlike those established for ambulatory care by an agreement between the government and the medical unions (Durand-Zaleski, Colin and Blum-Boisgard 1997).

[2] This agency replaces ANDEM (*Agence nationale pour le développement de l'évaluation médicale*), which was created in 1990 by the Ministry of Health to develop

and promote medical evaluation. ANDEM played an important role in organizing consensus conferences and the development of clinical guidelines.

[3] The AP-HP group comprises 50 hospitals, 28,000 beds, 84,000 nurses, 62,000 auxiliaries and 11,000 doctors, of which 850 are university professors.

References

Audeleley, G. R., P. Ravaud , B. Giraudeau, L. Kerboul, R. Nizard, P. Massin, C. Garreau de Loubresse, C. Vallée, and P. Durieux. 1997. Implementation of the Ottawa Ankle Rules in France. *Journal of the American Medical Association* 277:1935-9.

Bastuji-Garin, S., A. Shaeffer, P. Wolkenstein, B. Godeau, C. Carville, I. Durand-Zaleski, M. Meignan. 1998. Pulmonary embolism. Lung scanning interpretation: about words. *Chest* 114:1551-5.

Colin, C., and L. Geffroy. 1997. The health system: reform wanted by government and expected by patients. *The Lancet* 349:791-92.

Derry, J., and M. Lawrence. 1991. Auditing audits: the method of the Oxfordshire medical audit advisory group. *British Medical Journal* 303:1247-49

Donabedian, A. 1989. Institutional and professional responsibilities in quality assurance. *Quality Assurance in Health Care* 1:3-11

Durand-Zaleski, I., J. C. Rymer, F. Roudot-Thoraval, J. Revuz, and J. Rosa. 1993. Reducing unnecessary laboratory use with a new test request form. *The Lancet* 342:150-3

Durand-Zaleski, I., N. Vasile, F. Lemaire, S. Aubry, and G. Frija. 1994. Management audit in a Department of Radiology: the example of a French hospital. *Investigational Radiology*29:797-801.

Durand-Zaleski, I., R. Leclerq, M. Bagot, F. Lemaire, J. Revuz, Y. Spetebroodt, E. S. Zafrani, and H. Rochant. 1996. Making choices in hospital resource allocation: the use of an evaluation tool to decide which new programs are financed. *International Journal of Technology Assessment in Health Care* 12:163-71.

Durand-Zaleski, I., C. Colin, and C. Blum-Boisgard. 1997. An attempt to save money by using mandatory practice guidelines in France. *British Medical Journal* 315: 943-6.

Durieux, P., and P. Ravaud. 1997. From Clinical Guidelines to Quality Assurance: the experience of Assistance Publique-Hôpitaux de Paris. *International Journal for Quality in Health Care* 9:215-9.

Fontaine, A., P. Vinceneux, A. F. Pauchet Traversat, and C. Cathala. 1993. Toward quality improvement in a French hospital: structures and culture. *International Journal for Quality in Health Care* 9:177-81.

Henderson, A. 1982. The test request form: a neglected route for communication between the clinician and the clinical chemist? *Journal of Clinical Pathology* 35:986-8.

de Pouvourville, G. 1997. Quality of care initiatives in the French context. *International Journal for Quality Assurance in Health Care* 9:163-17

Shaw, C., and T. E. Brooks. 1991. Health service accreditation in the United Kingdom. *Quality Assurance in Health Care* 3:133-40.

Weingarten, S. 1978. Practice guidelines and prediction rules should be subject to careful clinical testing. *Journal of the American Medical Association* 277:1977-8.

Zaat, J., J. van Eijk, and H. Bonte. 1992. Laboratory test form influences test ordering by general practitioners in the Netherlands. *Medical Care* 30:189-92.

Chapter 7

Quality Management at the University of Pennsylvania Health System

David Shulkin and Maulik Joshi

The University of Pennsylvania Health System (UPHS) is an academic-based, integrated delivery system serving the populations of three states—Pennsylvania, New Jersey and Delaware. As a horizontally and vertically integrated health system, UPHS is composed of 4 owned hospitals (with over 1,700 total beds), 10 affiliated hospitals/health systems, 400 primary care physicians, 1,400 specialty physicians and services in behavioral health, skilled nursing, home care, long-term care, rehabilitation and hospice. On an annual basis, UPHS encounters over 70,000 inpatient admissions and 2 million outpatient visits.

Quality management in the American medical care system has a long history and has experienced a profound transformation over the last ten years. Traditionally, quality was addressed from an assurance perspective, focusing upon identifying outlier cases for improvement. The quality assurance (QA) function was typically acknowledged as a necessary, yet non-critical strategy in the delivery of optimal health care. Quality assurance was concentrated in the hospital setting and had a primary role in monitoring a collection of indicators to ensure compliance to regulatory and medical care standards. The common practice was to discover errors, identify the sources (the people or the process) and rectify the situation to prevent future problems.

In the 1980's, industrial management techniques of total quality management (TQM) or continuous quality improvement (CQI) began to take hold in health care. This approach brought a different philosophy and set of tools to the task of improving quality than have been traditionally applied (Chassin 1997; Berwick and Nolan 1998). Quality management embarked on a paradigm shift from an assurance to an improvement model. The new approach to quality had two distinct aspects. An increased focus upon systems and processes and their impact upon results and a more rigorous foundation in outcomes measurement. These scientific innovations had a dramatic effect upon the attitude of health care workers and organizations.

At Penn, quality management has followed a similar pattern, from an assurance, hospital-based model to one that is focused on improvement and the continuum of care. This redesign of the quality management function progressed in three stages. The first stage was a philosophical and cultural shift from an emphasis upon regulatory compliance and assessment to one of continuous improvement. Traditional quality assessment roles of data collection, routine assessment and preparation for regulatory and accreditation standards were de-emphasized. The expectations for quality management were now to proactively measure gaps in meeting customer needs or in providing optimal clinical care and to identify strategies to improve any deficiencies.

The second stage encompassed a change in the infrastructure of the quality program through the development of two programs: Clinical Resource Management (CRM) and Clinical Pathways and Quality Improvement Systems (CPQIS). The CRM program was designed to bring case-management services to the hospital environment, and as a result, to improve quality and reduce costs. The CRM program resulted in a new role of the clinical resource coordinator whose duties included collection of concurrent outcomes data, providing interventions to improve quality and efficiency and interacting directly with third party payers. The CPQIS Office was developed to support the development, implementation and evaluation of clinical pathways and practice guidelines as tools to reduce clinical practice variation. The professionals in this office focus upon identifying best clinical practices, incorporating those elements into pathways and having an infrastructure for collecting data elements and evaluating the impact of guidelines on outcomes such as patient satisfaction, clinical indicators such as complications, readmissions and mortality, length of stay and costs. The office is also responsible for oversight and dissemination of health and functional status assessment initiatives, as well as health risk assessment strategies.

Building upon the structure and success of the aforementioned programs, the final element of the continuum of care and service was the expansion of quality management to the Health System. This expansion shifted the emphasis away from solely an inpatient focus to the inclusion of initiatives in the primary care, home care, rehabilitation, long term care, behavioral health and hospice settings. This also provided an important opportunity to integrate care and improvement across multiple delivery settings, which lead to the creation of Penn Health and Disease Management (PHM). The objectives of PHM are to integrate primary care and specialty care quality services and measures in order to track outcomes for an episode of care of specific patient populations or disease categories. PHM goes beyond improving the care for patients who receive services when ill, to improving the health of a patient population.

With this evolution as background, the remainder of the chapter focuses upon a description of the major elements of Penn's quality management program and lessons learned from each of the critical areas.

The UPHS Quality Management Program

The UPHS Quality Management program is based on the following key principles:

A philosophy of doing the right thing at the right time in the right place;
Leadership that is committed to the quality management doctrine;
An organizational structure that supports quality improvement across the continuum of care;
A measurement system that provides data and information critical to improvement efforts;
Accountability at all levels of the organization to continuously improve; and
Diverse methods and tools of quality improvement.

Philosophy

Continuously improving the quality of care and service at UPHS is a fundamental element of the mission and vision of the Health System. The function of quality improvement is thus a responsibility of every individual who is a part of the Health System. A sound quality management philosophy is intricately linked to the organizational mission and vision, as evident from the following excerpt from the Health System Strategic Quality Management Plan:

"The University of Pennsylvania Health System strives to provide the highest quality of care in the region and the nation. UPHS's approach to quality improvement is designed in accordance with *our mission to create the Future of Medicine through education, research and the delivery of extraordinary care to the people of the greater Philadelphia region.* Our ultimate vision of success and the integral role of quality management is to implement a fully integrated academic health system providing the best possible care with the best possible service and the least possible hassle and least possible cost for our patients and other customers."The overall goals of quality management at UPHS include:

- To provide a consistent, high level of care and service to all patients in the most effective, appropriate and resource efficient manner.
- To provide a seamless, integrated level of service and care for patients within the Health System.
- To continuously improve outcomes related to the quality of patient care.
- To provide national leadership in the field of quality management through the development and dissemination of best practices.
- The structure and process surrounding these principles are essential components of an organizational culture of quality improvement. These goals serve as the basic tenets for all activities that strive to meet the goals of the organization.

Lessons Learned

To instill a true quality improvement philosophy into everyday practice, the principles of the program must be embedded in the organization's vision, mission and strategic priorities. The program goals must be clearly articulated and demonstrate that success of the organization hinges upon the success of continuous quality improvement. Additionally the program philosophy must be based on acknowledged factors that correlate highly to meaningful improvement. For example, quality at UPHS addresses the key drivers of success in meeting and exceeding customer needs by providing *easy access to great service, great quality of care and great value.* These drivers were identified based upon extensive market research that quantitatively and qualitatively examined the reasons why patients are retained by the organization or lost to other organizations.

Leadership

Organizing a system for improvement depends on effective leadership and on sophisticated understanding among physicians about why and how they can assist organizational leaders (Berwick and Nolan 1998). The quality improvement culture begins with the dedication of leadership to the program and the process. At Penn, this is achieved by the leadership of the Chief Quality Officer/Chief Medical Officer for the Health System, who reports directly to the Chief Executive Officer, and is responsible for quality management in the Health System, including oversight and implementation of clinical management strategies and quality measurement activities.

Leadership, however, extends beyond one individual accountable for the process. Leadership is evident through personal involvement of administrative and clinical managers in the quality improvement function. Involvement includes membership of improvement committees, participation in specific improvement project teams, or championing team recommendations by providing a supportive environment for testing interventions. Identified below are specific examples of quality management programs lead by different champions in the Health System.

A Senior Medical Director for Education in Quality directs a Managed Care and Quality Management course collaboratively designed by UPHS clinicians for physician faculty. This six-hour course is required for all new UPHS physician faculty, as well as physicians seeking re-appointment. The course is a highly interactive, case-based program designed to provide opportunities to share and learn on prevailing quality principles. For enhanced interaction, participants use a hand held audience response system to allow for real time survey question answers in a group setting. Course topics include outcome measurement development, financial risk management in managed care, clinical guideline development and implementation, clinical resource management, health promotion, disease management and cost-effectiveness analyses.

A senior medical director (with associate medical directors) directing the Penn Health and Disease Management program which entails the integration of best practices, patient education, provider protocols, clinical information support systems, case management, prevention and wellness, health risk appraisal, outcome measurements, demand management and quality improvement into comprehensive care programs.

A national physician fellowship program directed by the Chief Medical Officer that annually enrolls four to six physicians throughout the country to spend a year at UPHS to learn and lead quality improvement in the Health System. Experienced physicians spend the year at UPHS learning quality improvement principles through exposure and interaction with Health System leaders, educational classes and seminars, and active participation and direction of specific medical management programs.

The aforementioned programs are directed by individuals who are not dedicated to those efforts full-time, but practicing clinicians or senior managers who contribute to developing and implementing programs on a part-time basis.

Lessons Learned

A continuous improvement culture requires support and dedication of clinicians and administrators at all levels of the organization. Leadership support, however, is not limited to committee membership or participation on teams. Leadership is championing the products or results of team activities. Leadership's role is to create an environmental tension where change is the expectation and not the exception. Challenging the status quo and accelerating improvement projects are characteristics of effective management

At Penn, the role of leadership in the improvement process is evident in the success and failure of projects. The diffusion of project results to other areas and services is strongly correlated with leadership involvement. Administrators who champion the interventions and promote their successes to other individuals and departments serve as a catalyst in other adopting the better practices. Those projects that do not have clinical or administrator director champions have a greater hurdle in achieving lasting success.

Additionally at Penn, physician leaders have been effective in the quality movement because of their role as not solely administrators, but practicing physicians who contribute their time in both leading and supporting initiatives. Practicing physicians serving in these roles garner respect from their colleagues and lend credibility to the quality management program and increase the likelihood of acceptance of change in processes or behaviors.

Organizational Structure

Integration of quality management across a multi-facility, multi-service health system requires a structure that will facilitate quality improvement across entities (such as hospitals) and disciplines (for example, nurses and physicians). This integration is achieved through both individuals and groups or committees.

At Penn, the quality management function is representative of a coordinated, decentralized organizational structure. Quality management is implemented by the directors of quality at each individual institution as improvement is driven locally by the persons most knowledgeable about the structures and processes of a specific entity or service. However, strategic planning and resources are centralized at the corporate level to ensure efficiency in design and implementation. The quality management program is lead by the individual who serves as both the Chief Medical Officer and Chief Quality Officer whose role is that of oversight and implementation of clinical and quality management activities. Reporting directly to the Chief Quality Officer is the Senior Director of Quality, who is accountable for the consistency of care and service across entities in the Health System through coordination of the individual quality directors.

Composed of senior leadership, the UPHS Quality Management Oversight Committee is responsible for strategic planning and oversight of quality in the Health System and accountable to the Board of Trustees. Each entity in the Health System reports to one of three committees (Specialty Services, Inpatient and Outpatient), all of which ultimately report to the Quality Management Oversight Committee. The diagram below outlines the committee structure, which depicts the integration of Health System components and the relationship of working quality improvement committees or teams and oversight committees.

Within the hospital structure, an important structural change has been the development of a clinical service line quality improvement approach. The traditional method of quality improvement was through a departmental structure where departments reported on their activities to the organizational improvement committee. This was changed to a service or product line approach to emulate the process from the patient's perspective. The service line quality improvement committee approach has redefined the manner in which quality is addressed in the hospitals and the ambulatory physicians by replacing departmental quality improvement committees with a multidisciplinary effort. There are thirteen service line quality committees between the hospitals and the clinical practices (cardiac, cancer, geriatric, psychiatry, emergency, surgical, medicine, women and infants, liver and digestive, trauma, neurosciences, musculoskeletal, and pulmonary). The service line infrastructure is instrumental

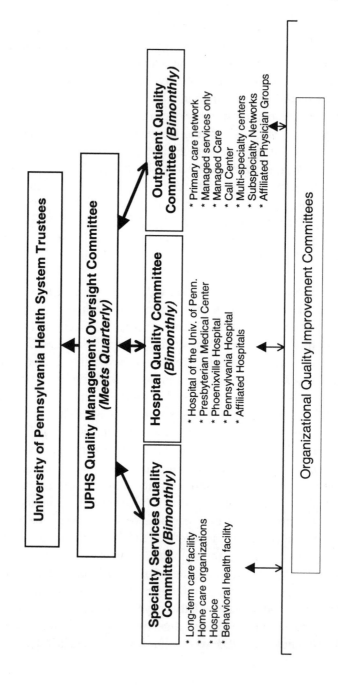

Figure 1. Organizational Structure of Quality Management

in quickly identifying improvement opportunities, designing and implementing interventions and evaluating changes in an integrated, comprehensive manner.

Lessons Learned

Avedis Donabedian and other quality pioneers have suggested that good structure increases the likelihood of good process, and good process increases the likelihood of a good outcome(Donabedian 1988). Structure, although only a part of the whole, is critical as it is the system in which processes and results occur. An effective structure includes:

All components of the medical care system;
Clinical and administrative leaders;
Empowered individuals at each organization to design and implement improvement; and
An individual and committee structure that is accountable for integrating and assuring quality care across multiple components

Measurement System

Key outcome measures at UPHS are monitored through the UPHS Scorecard Measurement and Improvement System (SMIS) that uses **Balanced Scorecards** to effectively and efficiently monitor performance at multiple levels. Balanced Scorecards operationalize strategic goals, focus upon the four key customer areas of service, clinical quality, access and value and are the foundation for the continuous improvement cycle. Additionally, the strategic planning process inherent in this measurement system provides the impetus for identifying, measuring and testing improvement initiatives. The objectives of this system are to:

Shift the paradigm from performance assessment to performance improvement;
Empower individuals and teams to manage their own critical processes based on data;
Establish organizational, team and individual accountability;
Set priorities and allocate resources;
Establish the link between the strategic imperatives of the organization,

the team and the individual as cascading bottom-up and top-down processes; and
Provide a balance between service, quality, access and value in the overall evaluation of performance.

Figure 2 depicts the role of the Scorecard Measurement and Improvement System in strategic planning and evaluation.

The UPHS SMIS is built upon the measurement of critical markers of an organization's success and the areas that demonstrate significant improvement opportunity. At the top level, UPHS Scorecards are integral for governance functions in terms of evaluation of overall performance, as well as monitoring of improvement activities. The CEO also reviews all the Scorecards monthly with the senior management team that consists of the chief and senior executives of the organization. The entity Scorecards (for example, the hospital) are discussed with the entity's management team (for example, associate administrators and clinical directors). The clinical and administrative directors then discuss their departments' Scorecard with their department directors. Ultimately, the department directors on an ongoing basis, discuss the department Scorecard with their staff for performance feedback. This process therefore ensures that communication loop is complete and the Scorecards are used at multiple levels for multiple objectives. A natural outgrowth of this process has been the collegial sharing and learning amongst front line managers of how programs and services are able to improve their measures, as evident on their Scorecards. Scorecards are shared at forums such as Department Directors Councils to provide a continuous quality improvement environment in striving to improve performance and achieving target goals.

Each UPHS Scorecard includes overall goals for the year and for each of the four dimensions of performance: service, quality, access and value. Measures have been developed from a bottom-up process and verified and audited for reliability and validity. Threshold, target and high performance goals are established for each measure based upon historical performance, trends and comparative benchmark data. Threshold goals are established so that they may be achieved with an improvement from baseline. Targets are established with the recognition that there must be significant improvement to achieve that level. As an example, the high performance goal is a 95% statistically significant improvement from baseline for a patient satisfaction measure.

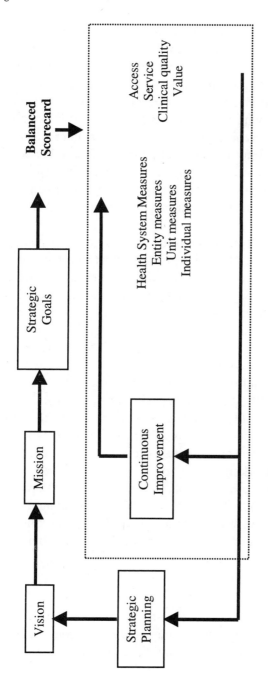

Figure 2. Scorecard Measurement and Improvement System

The UPHS Scorecards include measures impacted upon by strategic improvement initiatives that will benefit the department and subsequently the organization. As an example, the UPHS Scorecard for Infection Control includes measures of nosocomial infections and variance from budget, which directly impact the overall care provided and overall organizational costs. By focusing and improving the Scorecard measures for infection control, the department and the organization benefit. Support for improvement is provided not only by quality improvement staff, but also from other sources such as internal human resources performance consultants and management. Continuous quality improvement methods, workout sessions and re-engineering activities are thus integral tools in the implementation of improvement projects to achieve established goals.

The information system platform used to generate measurement and information is the foundation to the measurement and improvement process. The ultimate goal of access to real-time, comprehensive medical data will result from the implementation of an electronic medical record system. Penn is piloting such a system, however, it will be a few years until all the delivery components of the Health System will be connected. As with practically all health care organizations, the interim process will focus upon interfacing existing databases and systems.

UPHS utilizes multiple clinical decision support systems to integrate clinical, resource utilization and financial information for analysis. These systems provide the ability to analyze variance from clinical pathways, profile physicians, profile resource consumption across major diagnostic categories and identify improvement opportunities within the organization through internal and external benchmarking.

The UPHS information warehouse compiles all the clinical and claims data from the over 150,000 members of the full risk contract arrangements with local HMOs. This warehouse integrates billing, scheduling, utilization and quality elements into a single source of information providing significant accessibility and power to analyze a system of care.

Lessons Learned

Measurement is traditionally a double-edged sword as it can both enable and impede progress. A successful measurement system must be designed to be flexible in meeting the needs of multiple audiences (senior executives, department directors and staff) and serving multiple purposes (organizational management or program evaluation).

Scorecards help to reduce the tendency to react to only one or two measures at a time and encourage the recognition of other perspectives or a balanced approach to understanding processes and their impact upon multiple dimensions of performance. Scorecards heighten the understanding and interdependencies associated with actions that may result in tradeoffs of one metric for another— for example, cost for quality. Scorecards are essential ingredients of a successful improvement culture because of their ability to identify multiple goals, quantify their objectives and provide the framework to understand the impact of changes.

Measurement in itself is a motivator for improvement. However, comparison or benchmarking of data serves as a catalyst in the use of information for management and improvement. As a resource, the UPHS Corporate Quality Office maintains and routinely distributes a Benchmark Database that includes among its many elements, information on outstanding performance internally and externally in global measures (for example, overall satisfaction), as well as detailed indicators (such as, complication rates for specific DRGs). The Benchmark Database provides a first-line resource in identifying high performers, learning from their processes and establishing goals to reflect their improvement opportunity. In addition to databases, participation in national information systems provides additional value in comparative performance.

Accountability

Accountability for quality management is built upon the guiding principle that quality improvement is the job of every employee. Consequently, organizational quality goals were developed based upon strategic priorities. Table 1 contains the Quality Goals for the Health System for 1998 reflecting the diversity and comprehensiveness of responsibility for the delivery of high quality care to the communities we serve.

Building upon the Quality Goals and utilizing the Scorecard Measurement and Improvement System, financial incentives are linked to specific measures within each department's Scorecard. For example, an employee in a specific department has a financial incentive for the organization's overall measure in patient satisfaction and financial incentive measures for his/her department in quality and value. The individual is thus linked financially to the success of

SERVICE GOALS
Improve patient and family satisfaction in all settings (inpatient, outpatient, home) with targeted areas in satisfaction with the physician, the nurse, and office staff — *Achieve significant improvement at the 95% confidence level*
Improve satisfaction of the providers of care — *Achieve significant improvement at the 95% confidence level with physicians' overall satisfaction with the organization and their likelihood of recommending the organization to others for care*
CLINICAL QUALITY GOALS
Improve clinical indicators in the outpatient setting including measures in immunizations and cancer screenings — *Achieve scores equal to Healthy People 2000 national goals*
Improve clinical indicators in the inpatient setting including reducing mortality, infections, and adverse events — *Decrease rates by 10%*
Improve clinical indicators in other settings such as reducing pressure ulcers in long term care and reducing readmissions and complications in home care services — *Reduce rates by 10%*
Improve the continuity of care through appropriate referral practices
Improve the appropriateness of the site of care delivery — *Increase the use of the call center by 50%*
ACCESS GOALS
Improve access in the outpatient setting in specific areas of satisfaction with the appointment scheduling process, time until the appointment, waiting time in the office and referrals — *Achieve significant improvement at the 95% confidence level*
Improve access in the inpatient setting in the specific areas of admissions and discharge — *Achieve significant improvement at the 95% confidence level*
Improve satisfaction with receiving home care services as necessary — *Achieve significant improvement at the 95% confidence level*
Reduce wait times for services and referrals — *Reduce wait times for services by 10%*
Improve satisfaction with telephone use and the reduction of non-accommodated appointments — *Reduce non-accommodated appointments to 1% of all calls*
VALUE GOALS
Reduce costs associated with the processes of care and management of the risk populations — *Reduce $15 million in inpatient costs*
Attain appropriate length of stay — *Achieve severity-adjusted LOS to benchmark, comparable organizations*
Reduce the health risk behaviors of our population — *At a community level, increase the number of measures that achieve national goals for healthy behavior*
Improve the functional and health status of our population — *Improve scores from surveys such as the SF-12, SF-36 and disease specific instruments*

Table 1. Health System Quality Goals

the organization's patient service and the success of the department in achieving its quality and financial goals. The financial incentive measure promotes a "win-win-win" atmosphere, for as the department achieves its goals, so does the organization and so do the customers we serve.

For example, Scorecards are developed and used for each patient unit of the Hospital of the University of Pennsylvania (HUP). Data sources for the patient care units include patient satisfaction surveys, accounting and finance, pathway variance database, internal clinical outcomes databases, clinical decision support information systems, administrative datasets (for example, UB92) and incident reports. All patient satisfaction data are coded by the medical record number, allowing stratification of responses by diagnoses and the site of care. This level of detail provides information that is closer to the specific employee level. Employees of one nursing floor are thus reviewing information from their specific floor for which their performance can impact the scores directly. The table below identifies the measures analyzed by each patient unit with the asterisked measures representing the incentive compensation measures. The inclusion of measures such as the satisfaction with the room and accommodations and the discharge process indicate the multi-disciplinary team approach to the SMIS process. These measures require involvement from other departments (for example, housekeeping, facilities management and clinical resource management) in the review of this information at the patient unit level and the design of improvements to achieve performance goals.

The patient care unit Scorecards are discussed between staff and the nurse managers to review performance and discussed at nursing leadership forums between the manager and organizational leaders. The unit Scorecard represents a balanced perspective on the performance of their unit in support of the organization's mission and the incentive compensation measures linked to the Scorecard assure accountability for improvement.

Lessons Learned

Increasing the accountability for improvement of core processes in the medical care system is achieved through multiple pathways, one of which is financial incentives. This linkage is achieved at the organizational and team level. Employees are rewarded when the team. department and organizationsucceed as a whole. The next, critical step is to extend the dimension one level further

A. Service	B. Clinical Quality
1. Nursing attitude toward visitors	1. Patient Fall Rate (falls/1000 patient days)
2. Staff concern for privacy	2. Severe fall-related injury rate
3. Degree to which staff treated you with respect/dignity	3. Nosocomial Pressure Ulcer Rate
4. Nursing Overall	4. Nurses' sensitivity and responsiveness to pain
5. Nurses attention to special needs	5. Nurses information on tests
6. Staff sensitivity to inconvenience	6. Adequacy of advice for care at home
7. Overall Room/Accommodation	7. Nurses info re medications
8. *Service Excellence patient satisfaction**	8. Patient perception of technical skills
	9. Adequacy of info given to family
C. Access	D. Value
1. Nurses promptness	1. Specialty bed utilization (bed days)
2. Speed of admission	2. Expenses per patient day
3. Assistance with discharge arrangements	3. ALOS/Case Mix Index
4. Amount of notice you were given to plan for discharge	4. Variance from budget
	5. Pathway variance tool completion

Figure 3. Patient Care Unit Scorecard

to the individual. This will enhance shared accountability across each area. The link to compensation provides the strategic crossroads of the success of an organization built upon the success of the entity, the team and the individual.

A crucial element of the SMIS process is that the measures included on the Scorecard have been identified by the department through a bottom-up process. This process is paramount in having individuals and departments "own" the information and its use. The measures and goals are reviewed by the Corporate Quality office to ensure consistency in setting goals and the reliability and validity of the data. However, the process needs to be driven by staff in order for them to have the ability to impact the measures directly from their work.

Quality Management Methods and Tools

Quality management methods and tools encompass a wide range of products and services, including but not limited to pathways, guidelines, education and performance reports. UPHS has over 80 clinical management strategies (inpatient pathways, outpatient guidelines and disease management programs) in implementation throughout the Health System and an additional 40 in the developmental stage. At Penn, implementation of clinical pathways and health and disease management programs have been the two major programs designed to improve patient care outcomes. The reason for the implementation of these activities is threefold:

> The integration of the Health System with multiple owned hospitals and primary care practices provided an imperative to address clinical quality issues facing a patient at any point of the medical care process. A leadership mandate that increased efficiency, as determined by reduced costs and utilization, was not to be undertaken at the expense of quality and service. Thus, a balanced approach to measurement and improvement was integral to the implementation of the activities.

> Market research, patient focus groups and staff and provider feedback demonstrated the desire for providing a single, high quality standard of coordinated care for customers in the communities that we serve.

Clinical Pathways

The goals of the UPHS clinical guidelines are to help patients make evidence-based decisions about health care through shared decision-making, reduce unexplained variations in practice and serve as tools for improving health outcomes in a cost-effective manner. The UPHS clinical pathways consist of streamlined documentation requirements, automated pathway variance data, patient pathways, educational materials and standardized order sets.

The selection of the initial 30 areas for pathway development were based upon explicit criteria that identified gaps from best practices in terms of mortality, morbidity, complications, readmission rates, length of stay, cost and patient satisfaction; high volume areas and expressed interest by physicians or other stakeholders like payers.

As with most improvement efforts, the success of the project hinges upon the buy-in and leadership of clinical champions with support from quality improvement professionals. Multidisciplinary teams were formed for each pathway with a physician and nurse co-chair with the charge to search and identify best practices and outcomes nationally. This was performed through analysis of the data contained in the information systems, literature searches, networking with colleague institutions and formal site visits to other organizations. Support of the pathways teams is provided by the Director of Quality Improvement Systems and staffed by nurse pathway coordinators who support the team's activities quantitatively (through data collection and analysis) and qualitatively (facilitating team progress). The composition of the teams included physicians, nurses, clinical administrators and other practitioners as appropriate (such as, infectious disease, respiratory, pharmacy, laboratory).

Once draft pathways were developed, the pathways were implemented in selected areas to test their compliance and effectiveness. Data were reported from the scannable variance tools (one page survey instruments to be completed by the providers throughout the course of patient's stay that document test results and treatment compliance), patient satisfaction and clinical and cost information. Patient satisfaction data are collected through an inpatient survey that is coded by each patient's medical record number. We thus have the ability to stratify all data by patients and are able to compare the satisfaction of patients on pathways versus those not on pathways. Clinical data are collected through administrative systems, as well as concurrently by clinical resource coordinators who collect over 20 data elements during a patient's stay (for example, infection, adverse event, medication error, return to ICU, readmission). The data are collected and communicated to the pathway team on an ongoing basis to review and refine the programs as necessary. Communication to all staff is also important as a performance feedback mechanism and posterboards are developed to communicate the key interventions and findings for each pathway. Data are also benchmarked nationally to identify not only longitudinal improvement, but also for comparison with other peer organizations.

As an example, the table below demonstrates solely the value impact of a sample of nine pathways at HUP that has resulted in a charge savings of over eight million dollars.

Pathway	Baseline LOS*	Post-implementation LOS	Charge Differential (US $)
Carotid Endarterectomy	5.2	3.2	2,299,950
Laparascopic Cholecystectomy	3.3	2.8	184,000
Renal Transplant	14.8	8.7	3,369,410
Radical Prostatectomy	4.9	3.4	1,250,690
Total Hip Replacement	7.9	5.8	727,000
Radiculopathy	5.0	3.5	1,683,300
Cardiac Angioplasty	4.3	3.6	(2,440,200)
Total Abdominal Hysterectomy	5.4	4.3	1,047,750
Craniotomy	10.5	9.1	308,205
Total Savings			**8,430,105**

*Length of stay

Table 2. Financial Impact of Clinical Pathways

Health and Disease Management

Health and disease management may be defined as a clinical improvement process aimed at ensuring that the best practices known to medical science are incorporated with minimal variation over the entire continuum of care (Todd and Nash 1996). The Penn Health and Disease Management (PHM) program coordinates resources throughout the organization in partnership with patients, clinicians, payers, vendors and other providers to enhance patient care outcomes. PHM programs encompass coordinated services consisting of clinical guidelines, physician and patient education, health risk assessment, case management, preventive care and wellness activities.

PHM programs address many characteristics that are major causes of poor quality and high cost in health care. Listed below are some of the barriers or deficiencies in the medical care system and the targeted interventions PHM programs utilize to address each cause:

- *Cause: The failure to prevent disease* PHM: Initiate and emphasize health screening and disease prevention programs

- *Cause: Failure to follow "best practices"* PHM: Ensure implementation of best practices through clinical guideline development and use, provider education, patient education and utilization of case managers and home health professionals
- *Cause: High risk patients* PHM: Identify high risk patients early through risk assessment programs, claims and encounter data
- *Cause: Non-compliance* PHM: Improve compliance through education, enhanced provider-patient contact and use of case managers and home health professionals
- *Cause: Late diagnosis of acute disease* PHM: Promote early disease recognition, diagnosis and treatment by patient education and provider

Lack of coordination of services and programs for patients and the use of best practices as documented through multiple data sources (including feedback from patients in satisfaction surveys and focus groups) was a significant impetus for the development of PHM programs.

Each PHM program includes, specific outcome indicators, patient education materials, provider educational materials, health risk appraisals and customized health and physical forms. Most programs also include case management for moderate and high-risk patient as determined by the stratification from the health risk appraisal system, which uses disease specific instruments, as well as standardized instruments such as the PRA, SF-12, nutritional screening and the Health Status Questionnaire. A new model of case management is being developed and tested as disease-specific "care managers" are working with patients one-on-one and in group sessions by disease to provide an additional resource to the physician's care of the patient population. These focused care managers provide significant experience and expertise in chronic conditions that require intensive education and management in modifying life-style behaviors and ensuring compliance to treatment protocols.

Ten programs are developed a year for a goal of 40 programs in place by the year 2000 which will cover 80% of all patient visits in the Health System. The first few programs include adult and pediatric asthma, diabetes, congestive heart failure, low back pain, hypertension, lipid management, smoking cessation, sleep apnea, weight management and osteoporosis.

Each Penn Health Management program team has an administrator, a clinical champion and a case manager with support from a data manager, a health and wellness director, a health risk appraisal director and a quality director. Additionally, clinical involvement is a must and includes primary and specialty physicians, nurses, office staff, physician extenders and ancillary support such as nutritional counselors, social workers, pharmacists and therapists. From the initial convening of the group to the pilot phase, over 20 individuals are involved in the development process, spanning all clinical and administrative functions, which occurs over a 3 month period. As a true CQI process, team members sign on "for life" in implementing and routinely evaluating and improving the programs based on new research and clinical innovations.

Health risk appraisal (HRA) studies provide a mechanism to continuously assesses the risks of the populations it serves and provides health and disease management interventions dependent upon the risk stratification categories. Using accepted, reliable and valid health risk questionnaires (for example, the SF-12, the HSQ, the PRA+), HRAs provide both a population perspective on health and provide feedback information to individuals on health risk behaviors. For the high-risk category, individuals may be contacted by case management experts, as well as be enrolled in specific health and disease programs. For the moderate risk group, information regarding specific resources and educational materials are shared. In all instances, the personalized profiles are shared with the primary care physician and the patient. The schematic below depicts the health and disease management interventions based upon health risk assessments.

All primary care practices that implement PHM programs are provided computers that include patient education software, as well as intranet access to all the programs. These multi-faceted programs are the culmination of identifying known best practices and translating those critical change elements into medical practice with enhanced support from other resources to provide optimal care for the patient in the most appropriate setting by the most appropriate provider. In addition to the speed of development and implementation of the program, clinical innovations such as emerging technology, new pharmaceuticals and new research are rapidly incorporated into the best practice disease management programs and diffused throughout the Health System both electronically and through dialogue with the clinical champions.

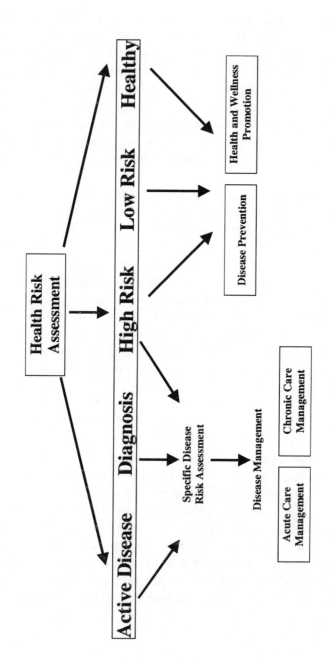

Figure 4. Health Risk Assessment

The success of physician involvement in quality improvement is evident not only in the results and impact on better patient outcomes, but also the increased satisfaction and desire on the part of physicians to participate and lead medical care redesign processes. For example, survey data yields that 95% of Penn physicians desire further participation in the Penn Health and Disease Management programs. A satisfaction survey of physicians also shows that from 1995 to 1997, there were statistically significant increases in the physician's overall satisfaction with the organization, their commitment to quality improvement and their perception of the quality of care provided by the organization.

Identified in the table below are clinical outcomes achieved to date on a sample of programs:

Lessons Learned
Health care quality improvement is based upon the fundamental principle of testing and evaluating new interventions in an effort to improve the medical delivery system. Guidelines, whether in the inpatient or outpatient setting, provide a consistent standard of care based on evidence of high performance. The pathway and disease management programs extend beyond clinical guidelines in attempting to improve clinical effectiveness across the continuum of care.

The success of developing and using clinical pathways rests upon fundamental quality improvement methods and tools. The development process included multiple individuals from diverse backgrounds to facilitate the buy-in of the process and included significant clinical leadership in championing the work of the teams. The emphasis was upon implementing evidence-based best practices and using outcomes data to document improvement in the care of the patients. Data was easily collected and communicated to the teams on an ongoing basis and refinements were made to emphasize the continuous improvement cycle. Additionally, pilot testing and the rapid diffusion of the early successes throughout the organization accelerated the use of the pathways and the ultimate improvement of patient care. The emphasis of the programs is also one of a quality improvement clinical strategy requiring a balanced focus on outcome measures.

Analogous to the key criteria for using inpatient pathways, the health and disease management programs focus upon central quality improvement

Measure	Improvement	Before	After
Asthma — Hospitalization rate	62% decrease	111 per 1,000	42 per 1,000
Asthma — % of patients with fewer than 2.4 days missed from work/school	66% decrease	67%	96%
Diabetes — % of patients with glycosylated hemoglobin <=8.0	50% increase	40%	60%
Diabetes — % of patients with ideal blood sugar levels	30% increase	51%	66%
CHF* — Hospitalization rate	96% decrease	532 per 1,000	21 per 1,000
CHF — Readmission rate	100% decrease	120 per 1,000	0 per 1,000
CHF — ER visit rate	69% decrease	255 per 1,000	80 per 1,000
CHF — % of patients on ACE Inhibitors	23% increase	70%	87%
Hypertension — % of patients with blood pressure <=140//<=90	179% increase	19%	53%

*Congestive heart failure

Table 3. Clinical Outcomes

principles. The development process included multiple individuals from diverse backgrounds to facilitate the buy-in of the process and included significant clinical leadership in championing the work of the teams. Involvement of both community-based physicians and academic specialty physicians integrate complimentary expertise and skills. Having the ability to customize programs for each primary care practice provides the dynamic flexibility necessary for successful implementation. Having available the essential resources for patients in the continuum of care (for example, case management and home care) is vital prior to coordinating the program.

The Future of Quality Management

The field of quality management in the health care industry continues to evolve at a rapid pace. The impetus for this accelerated progress is increased demand by payers (state and federal government, employers and ultimately consumers) to improve the care and services received from health care organizations. Quality management faces increased scrutiny and will need to continue to advance exponentially.

For quality management to be successful in this environment, a number of crucial elements must be in place. First and foremost, there must be buy-in from medical and administrative leadership on the value of investing resources in this field. There must also be increased rigor for reliable and valid measurement and evaluation of quality improvement activities. This lack of rigor in evaluation, a necessary element of quality improvement, has spurred the growth of a new industry called outcomes measurement.

Measurement, however is merely one component of the performance improvement process, as feedback of data and accountability for results complete the improvement cycle. Successful quality management programs are not separate from the daily operations of the organization, but are integrated within the core functions. At Penn, quality improvement is a part of the organizational mission and values and is the responsibility of every Health System employee, with a financial linkage to the performance of individuals, departments and the entire organization. An improvement culture is one that does not require a common quality improvement nomenclature or the use of an identical improvement model, but one in which the practice of improvement is supported, encouraged and expected.

Recently, the Institute of Medicine, a component of the National Academy of Sciences, issued a consensus statement on the "Urgent Need to Improve Health Care Quality." The statement noted that although considerable efforts and resources have been dedicated to quality improvement over the last two decades, serious and widespread quality problems exist throughout American medicine. To accomplish major, systematic improvement, there must be a major overhaul in how we deliver health care services, educate and train clinicians, and assess and improve quality (Chassin, Galvin and The National Roundtable on Healthcare Quality 1998). These revolutionary approaches are available, as we often know what the best practices are; however, it is the execution of these approaches that defines success.

References

Berwick, D. M., and T. W. Nolan. 1998. Physicians as Leaders in Improving Health Care. *Annals of Internal Medicine* 128(4):289-92.

Chassin, M. 1997. Assessing Strategies for Quality Improvement. *Health Affairs* 16(3):158-65.

Chassin, M. R., R. H. Galvin, and The National Roundtable on Healthcare Quality. 1998. The Urgent Need to Improve Health Care Quality. *Journal of the American Medical Association* 280 (11):1000-5.

Donabedian, A. 1988. The Quality of Care. *Journal of the American Medical Association* 260(12):1743-8.

Todd, W. E., and D. Nash. 1996. *Disease Management: A Systems Approach to Improving Patient Outcomes*. American Hospital Publishing Inc.: Chicago.

Part III. Potential

Chapter 8

Evaluating Quality Outcomes Against Best Practice: A New Frontier

Jon Chilingerian

Throughout the world, leaders in health care systems understand that improving quality on a *continuous* basis requires an ability to identify providers and facilities with the best results in practice. To this end, health care organizations in most developed countries have committed to adopting quality management programs and practices aimed at measuring and evaluating care provided and outcomes achieved (de Pouvourville 1997; Kenagy et al. 1999; Davies and Crombie 1997). The need to develop better measures of quality health services has convincingly been set forth by researchers (Brook et al. 1996).

Arguably, the measurement of quality is one of the most complex problems facing health care management today. For purposes of measurement, quality care cannot be determined by relying on clinical judgment alone. There are several assessment methods that look at care from various angles that should be considered, such as: the adequacy of care; outcomes achieved in relation to potential outcomes; actual service process in relation to standard process criteria; and results achieved in relation to prior expectations. These assessments should be applied to each of the four major tasks of health care delivery: (1) screening, (2) prevention, (3) diagnosis, and (4) treatment (Brook et al. 1996).

Another problem is deciding what types of decision-making units and at what levels of aggregation quality is to be measured. The complex architecture of clinical decision-making units begins with physicians (and/or care-providers) and patients, and aggregates into departments and facilities operating in multiple regions in a country. At the facility level, each of the decision-making units contains many different, independent types of providers, including: long term care, sub-acute care, rehabilitation, acute care, ambulatory care, and specialty care facilities. These units, which form neither a hierarchy nor a homogeneous set, confound the measurement of overall quality. Consequently, there is no uniform and hierarchical reporting system.

A third major problem in quality measurement is validity. To measure quality validly requires a deep knowledge of these clinical decision-making units and their activities, as well as some method that answers questions such as: how to group them, how they interact, how they are related to each other, and how they respond to data by changing their behavior. Research suggests that evidence of a high quality service for one activity, diagnosis, or symptom, cannot be generalized. High performers in one diagnosis or procedure might be average or below average in another diagnosis or procedure. Given the variety of assessment methods available, lack of uniform reporting systems, and the problem of validity, deriving comparative cross-national measures of quality remains an elusive and quixotic goal.

The point being made here is not that *quality* is too ambiguous, too formidable, or too complex to measure; the fact remains that having been given such a forbidding task, great progress has been made. In some systems such as France, Sweden, the United States, and Canada, payers, health plans, government policy-makers, competing providers, patient-activists, and other stakeholders (like the media) have become the driving force to promote quality of care. Although comprehensive quality improvement programs were first developed for acute care hospitals, today virtually every provider and care unit is making quality improvements (Meisenheimer 1997). Progress has taken place at several levels of decision making units—the physicians, the maternity wards, the hospitals, and nursing care facilities. These quality management programs would benefit from novel or improved analytic methods aimed at developing sound quality measures.

The focus of this chapter is on a new methodology to meet the challenge and difficulty of evaluating quality outcomes. It is argued that a methodology for quality measurement is needed that can accomplish several objectives:

(1) focus on individual observations (in contrast to provider averages);

(2) produce a single, overall measure as opposed to multiple measures;

(3) handle multiple indicators of quality, without knowledge of weights; and

(4) identify the units with the best outcomes and the magnitude of departure from best practices.

Traditional approaches to assess performance have focused on the central tendency of a cloud of statistical data points, without paying much attention to the extremes. Since extreme values are connected to small probabilities, central tendency theory considers extreme values to be outliers or errors. Although statistical analyses often ignore the outliers, studies of performance suggest that when measured correctly, some outliers can be interpreted as having achieved 'excellence' or a 'best practice' (Lewin and Minton 1986). Aside from Poisson's law, there have been few methodological developments in the acceptance and rejection of outlying values (Gumbel 1958). Data envelopment analysis (DEA) has the potential to be such a methodology (see Charnes et al. 1994).

DEA is introduced as a tool to profile and evaluate best practice outcomes. The orientation of DEA on analyzing the "best results observed in practice" and optimizing the clinical decision making unit has the potential to offer a new approach to quality measurement. In contrast to statistical approaches that focus on the "average" quality behavior, DEA calculates a quality measure for each clinical unit with the requirement that each unit being evaluated lie either on or below the quality-outcome frontier.

Although the main purpose of this chapter is to illustrate a new quality measure, the paper begins by making some conceptual distinctions necessary to understand quality measurement as a multi-dimensional construct. The first section explores the problem of measuring quality in a multi-dimensional problem. Based on the recent literature, each of five dimensions of quality will be discussed. These ideas will be illustrated on nursing home data from the United States. By tracing the improvements and deterioration in the functional status of a group of nursing home patients with DEA, an outcome frontier is identified and analyzed. The chapter ends with a discussion of why the quality movement would benefit from a methodology aimed at a identifying a best practices frontier and deriving measures accordingly.

Toward a Multi-Dimensional Definition of Clinical Quality: A Look at the Five Leading Dimensions

Throughout the 20th century, the *ostensible challenge* in health care management, was to find a theoretically correct way to assess quality of care; but the *real challenge* was uncovering and understanding some of the many factors underlying quality. While philosophical arguments have seldom delayed business leaders from finding solutions to practical, bottom-line problems, philosophical debates in health care among policy-makers, clinical leaders and managers have hindered the measurement of quality.

If there was a widely accepted, operational definition of quality of care, the measurement of quality would be somewhat simpler. However, the range of alternative routes to quality measurement takes us to very different places. For example, in the United States, the Institute of Medicine defines quality as "the degree to which health services for individuals and populations increase the likelihood of desired health outcomes and are consistent with current professional knowledge" (Chassin and Glavin 1998). Some health care systems, like Apollo Hospital System in India, defines quality in terms of "outstanding value to the patient," which not only means being discharged home, without morbidity, or mortality, but also finding the "quicker routes to health" with lower total costs (Chilingerian 1992). From a patient perspective *quality of care* means at first "not feeling well and then, after receiving care, feeling much better," which implies a capacity to achieve clinical satisfactory results (Steffan, 1988).

If quality could be treated as uni-dimensional variable, some subjective means of combining multiple measures (or a theory-based mathematic able to derive single, summary measure of quality) could be applied. For example, if variables such as mix of staff, methods of peer review, decision-making efficiency, convenience, patient satisfaction, health status, and mortality were highly inter-related, it would be possible to develop a single concept based on the general features or common elements of quality.[1] During this century, managers and policy-makers came to understand that quality could never become a simple concept.

This was, of course, one of the many important lessons that business management learned from the economists. Since individuals have widely diverging tastes and preferences, there could never be a "one best way" to assess the quality of services (Hemenway 1984). The assessment of service quality is always subjective—people will weight and rank the characteristics of services in inconsistent ways. Absent a guiding theory of quality, and at best we can identify some critical features, components, or underlying dimensions of quality, rank (or grade) them, and report the results. In this sense, measuring quality requires evaluating performance from a multidimensional scheme.

In health care, the multi-dimensionality of quality, has been recognized. Donabedian (1988) identified multiple levels to assess quality in terms of three categories: structure, process, and outcomes. Each one of those categories could include hundreds of variables.

There are multiple and conflicting outcome measures (ranging from indicators of changes in functional and health status to post-surgical infection and mortality rates), multiple clinical inputs (related to diagnosis and treatment), and qualitative factors such as "global" measures of patient satisfaction and time spent waiting. The measurement problem is confounded, not only by the multi-dimensional environment of quality, but also by the difficulty of measuring each of these dimensions of quality. Each dimension encompasses more than one underlying variable. The most promising direction is to assume that quality is not as complex as the vast enumeration of variables and indicators from the literature. Quality, as a construct, is best understood in terms of a few underlying dimensions.

According to the literature, at least five important dimensions of quality have emerged. These five dimensions can be seen in Table 1. They are: (1) patient satisfaction; (2) information and emotional support; (3) amenities/ convenience; (4) decision-making efficiency; and (5) outcomes. Although there is scant evidence to suggest that these five underlying dimensions are highly inter-correlated; they are not independent factors. Each dimension will be discussed.

Patient Satisfaction

Recently, as the orientation to health care began shifting from scientific mandates and medical techniques to markets and the more human side of health care, a service delivery system, *patient satisfaction* became an important dimension of quality of care (Gold and Wooldridge 1995; Berwick 1996). In part, the discovery of patient satisfaction was an artifact of clinical work on patient-centered care (Delbanco 1992) and the influence of strategic marketing on health care management. Clinicians learned that throughout the service process, patients and their families would experience hundreds of "clinical moments of truth." Research on the *satisfied patient* suggested that patients' overall evaluation of quality depend on the results of the processes as an "experience" at every point of contact.[2] Quality measurement, from this perspective, requires mapping and surveying the patient's entire experience with the delivery system.

Patient Satisfaction
– % extremely satisfied and why
– pain management
– % willing to recommend provider/use again
Information & Emotional Support
– amount and clarity of information
– time spent listening
– time spent encouraging
Amenities and Convenience
– clean, fast, accurate, timely
– patient treated with respect
– service available when needed
Decision-Making Efficiency
– clinical resources utilized to achieve constant quality outcomes
– quick routes to health (diagnosis, treatment)
Outcomes
– mortality/morbidity rates
– changes in functional status, health status and illness severity

Table 1. Five Leading Dimensions of Quality of Care

Performing medical care tasks produces valuable patient services, and feelings of satisfaction and dissatisfaction develop. Feelings of satisfaction are about meeting and exceeding patient/customer expectations (Hesket, Sasser and Schlesinger 1997). On the other hand, dissatisfaction may be related to the rate of uncertainty reduction throughout the care process (Schauffler and Rodriguez 1996). There are many different indicators of patient satisfaction, ranging from the patient's overall experience, to a patient's willingness to use and recommend the service in the future. To understand the patient's overall experience, there are several questions to pose: Were the patients treated rudely? Did they expect less waiting? Did they experience unnecessary uncertainty? Was there a focus on the patient, as an individual? Was the medication dosage too weak or too strong?

Although defection rates (the percentage of patients who change providers) are sometimes used (Struebing 1996), some critics suggest avoiding global measures of quality and focusing on the specific sources of satisfaction and dissatisfaction that might cause a defection. For example, rather than report a

90% satisfaction rate, report that 10 percent of the patients were dissatisfied because their physician never told them what to do or what not to do after they left the hospital and went home (Delbanco 1992). Patient information about extraordinarily good and bad services is captured in satisfaction. To avoid losing this information, patient satisfaction should be included in the medical record so all caregivers can regularly monitor each patient's experiences during the service encounters.

Although patient satisfaction is a critical dimension, the knowledge difference between patients and health care providers is so large that *substantial client satisfaction* cannot be the only indicator of quality. The practice of medicine contains "hidden actions" and equivocal information, so it is difficult for most patients to know whether diagnostic tests and other treatments were appropriate, and the outcomes reasonable. Therefore, measures of quality from other vantage points are required to review whether or not the process was adequate and the outcomes acceptable.[3] For these reasons, information and emotional support and amenities/convenience are included as separate dimensions.

Information and Emotional Support

The second dimension of quality is *information and emotional-support*. Although related to satisfaction, it is treated separately because it gives rise to another fundamental expectation in health services—increasing (or perhaps even optimizing) the patient's control. Good clinical care necessitates task-oriented provider behavior focused on diagnosing symptoms, setting treatment goals, and monitoring recovery. However, quality care also requires large amounts of relationship provider behavior on behalf of promoting the involvement of the individual and family, as well as informed choice, encouragement, clarification, and confidentiality.

When people are sick, patients and their families need to receive excellent care. They also need to have their voices heard and to feel supported and encouraged That is, they need empathy not sympathy. Some questions to pose are: To what extent do caregivers educate and clarify the treatment regimes, as well as spend time listening and encouraging? Was the examination thorough? Were patients told when and how to take their medications and what to eat? Are illnesses discussed not only with privacy in mind, but tactfully as well? To what extent was the diagnosis, results and care plan explained? While some of these factors may be measured by patient surveys, others should be based on audits of the medical records.

Some would argue that caregivers who involve patients and families in decisions, coach patients and give emotional support, reduce uncertainty— the clinical experience becomes manageable and less frightening. Benner (1984) reports that teaching patients to prepare before surgery can actually expedite their recovery. In fact, research suggests that providing better patient information and more effective emotional support can lead to shorter stays, less medication, fewer side effects, better compliance, and higher levels of satisfaction (Picker Report 1992).

Convenience of Care/Amenities

This third important dimension of quality of care reflects an individual patient's preferences for technology, people, facilities, and behaviors. Measuring these variables implies discovering choices among courses of clinical action and clinical decision making. While Donabedian (1988) has argued that "convenience, comfort, quiet, and privacy" are merely desirable attributes of the health care delivery system (p 1744); receiving care conveniently (and in a timely manner) might even be more important to some patients than achieving better clinical outcomes.

Herzlinger (1998) has argued that there are two new market segments or new consumers: people who want convenience; and people who demand more information. Today's hard working patients lead busy lives and increasingly will be demanding (and be deserving) of convenient and comfortable access to medical services. A growing number of surgeries can be substituted for a non-invasive version. Throughout Europe, for example, there are non-invasive centers for breast, brain, and heart therapy. Some patients need information regarding these new choices and their availability.

An argument could be made that amenities/convenience will be an integral part of any measure of patient satisfaction. If so, then why place them in separate dimensions? Amenities/convenience have been separated from overall patient satisfaction for two reasons. First, researchers have reported that when patients have been asked about their overall satisfaction, patients do not emphasize aesthetics, better food and parking, amenities and convenience (Delbanco 1992). Since individual tastes differ, the value of convenience depends on individual needs and preferences. These are culturally weighted preferences.

Another reason that amenities/convenience should be a separate dimension of quality is that service inconveniences have opportunity cost implications for patients, and offerings of greater convenience have cost implications for caregivers. As health care becomes increasingly competitive, trade-offs may be necessary to *stem* the health care cost explosion. By measuring this dimension separately, clinicians can be convinced of its importance; patients can be convinced when there is added-value. If the delivery system decides to make the service more convenient in a way that has value to a patient, a higher reimbursement or price can be charged.

Decision-Making Efficiency

A fourth dimension of quality can be called d*ecision-making efficiency* (Chilingerian and Sherman 1990; Chilingerian 1992), which is the least-developed of the five dimensions of quality and perhaps the most controversial. In the past, physicians were trained to do everything possible for the patient regardless of cost; moreover, physicians would equate more intensive medical care with better services. As Harris (1977) explains, "doctors have an almost inexhaustible repertoire of things that will make patients better off..." But what does 'better off' really mean? Providing superior clinical service today requires rapid information processing for diagnosis and treatment. There is growing evidence that quick and accurate diagnosis that expedites treatment increases a patient's chances of success, by reducing cycle times for hospitalization, recovery, follow-up treatment, and returning to a 'normal' life.

Since it makes no sense to evaluate the efficiency of a medical service process that results in morbidity, mortality, or a re-admission to a hospital, decision making efficiency must focus on the resources used in order *to achieve a satisfactory outcome*. Inefficiency in the provision of clinical services occurs when physicians and other care providers use an excessive amount of resources to achieve a satisfactory result. The over-utilization of medical services not only carries patient risks, but also increases patient anxiety. Moreover, some evidence exists that too many tests, needles, and x-rays may do more harm than good (Eisenberg 1986).

Outcomes[4]

This fifth dimension of quality, expresses the degree to which the observed clinical performance approached its potential. As one physician argued, "quality is not how well or how frequently a medical service is given, but how closely the result approaches the fundamental objectives of prolonging life, relieving distress, restoring function, and preventing disability. Important thinkers in health care have argued that outcomes are the leading indicator of quality, and the outcomes of greatest significance would be changes in health status attainable given current technology, clinical knowledge, and management practices.

Though outcomes vary considerably among clinical providers and systems of care, comparing the outcomes of health care providers can be difficult. Various reasons are put forth to explain outcome variations such as, prior health status, poor patient compliance, lack of diffusion of medical technology, poorly coordinated care, lack of competence of providers, weak clinical leaders, and ineffective management practices. According to Donabedian, outcomes record the effects of the care process on the health status of the population (1988). Outcomes include serious clinical results such as death, medication errors, post-operative loss of an organ or limb, or even a hospital-acquired infection. Measures can focus on the major clinical benefits that have actually been achieved, or focus on small improvements in-patient functioning along with disease specific clinical results.

The development of case-mix measures and/or indicators of health status, functional improvement, and severity of illness has advanced considerably. When case-mix measures are available, it is possible to develop summary measures of the clinical benefits achieved based on changes in functional status or other measures of patient outcomes (Chilingerian 1995). For example, measuring the change in severity of illness for a given diagnosis from admission to discharge would be a very good measure of effectiveness of the care process in attaining outcomes in relation to implied clinical objectives. How improvements or deterioration in patient outcomes can be incorporated into models of performance is the subject of the next section.

From Statistical Averages to Quality-Outcome Frontiers

One thorny problem facing clinical researchers seeking to measure quality outcomes is to wade through the vast literature. If good measures exist, there is no need to construct perfect measures. Though many measures do exist; few methodologies have been able to handle noncommensurate, multiple indicators of superior outcomes. There are also several weaknesses with traditional approaches to outcome measurement. So the question remains; are their new ways to think about measuring outcomes?

The outcome dimension of quality denotes the degree to which a service provider's observed performance achieves its potential. In order to assess performance success or improvements, outcome quality requires a performance standard or benchmark against which success can be measured. Deploying a benchmark or performance standard requires identifying a goal. However, it is possible to define goals in one of two ways: (1) achieving better than average outcomes; or (2), achieving the maximum obtainable (or best possible) outcomes observed in practice by service providers.

In the first case, standards are based on average performance outcomes of a frequency distribution of providers. The most common of the various methods used to study average performance is statistical analysis. For example, averages such as the mean mortality rates, medication error rates, infection rates, and other morbidity rates, attempt to convey the "central tendency" of a single ratio of a group of providers. Variations from mean rates are taken as worth identifying, and the standard deviation is a useful way to describe how far providers depart from the mean. Mean outcomes can be regressed in an ordinary least squares (or other) model to provide a measure of the proportion of variance in average performance outcomes that can be explained by other variables.

In the second case, standards are defined in terms of providers who have achieved the *best possible outcomes*. One measures quality by rank ordering providers based on their proximity or distance from an empirical (or relative as opposed to absolute) frontier. [5] Failure to attain outcomes near or at the frontier is assumed to be an important research question for health care management. In this case, once a standard such as, "achieving best outcomes" is established, optimization with respect to that objective will identify a *quality frontier*.

There are three weaknesses with the current methods of analyzing quality outcomes. The first problem with the current analytic measures is the reliance on a multitude of single rates and ratios. Since some rates will be high and some will be low, there is neither a sense of the overall degree of excellence achieved, nor an understanding of whether better results are even possible.

A second problem is that current analytic methods are directed at the central tendencies of health care providers, rather than the "best results observed in practice." Traditional assessments of quality outcomes have defined the performance standard based on achieving better than average outcomes and have not developed methods aimed at identifying the best possible outcomes. There is little doubt that measures of central tendency and variability are indispensable tools in quality measurement. As was pointed out above, however, studies of performance that identify central tendencies might yield weak and misleading information. In health care, significant comparisons should not be based on prevailing practice standards or norms based on the average behavior of providers over time. Since averaging profiles will not pinpoint how an individual physician or a health facility achieved their results, health care providers should benchmark their performance to the best in the delivery system.

A third weakness with current methods is that if each dimension of quality requires a battery of ratios and measures, quality measurement will be hopelessly lost in a sea of mythical averages as standards. Identifying departures from average performance by relying on multiple indicators for multiple dimensions will never produce an accurate picture of quality.

Frontier analysis shifts the focus from a hypothetical standard based on averages to those providers who actually did achieve the best outcomes. Identifying an *empirical quality frontier* limits the range of possible outcomes to what happened in practice. Outcomes observed below the quality frontier (providers who have achieved outcomes that are less successful than the best) are deficient. Since no providers will be observed above the frontier, providers at or near the frontier have achieved the "best results observed in practice." In short, the proximity or distance that a provider lies below the quality frontier can be regarded as a robust measure of outcome quality.

The task at hand is to translate the previous discussion on outcomes into a framework that not only identifies a quality frontier, but also permits estimation of the magnitude of departure from an empirical frontier. The most general method for deriving frontiers and measuring proximity from frontiers is data envelopment analysis (DEA), pioneered by Charnes, Cooper, and Rhodes (1978) and discussed in the next section.

Measuring Outcome Quality with Data Envelopment Analysis (DEA)
DEA is a methodology developed in the late 1970's for evaluating the "relative" performance of comparable decision making units (DMU) in multidimensional

space (see Charnes et al. 1994). Although most applications of DEA have been applied to estimations of technical efficiency and production frontiers, the methodology offers an empirical way to estimate various best practice frontiers. For example, any dimension of quality can be assessed by employing multiple indicators in a DEA model and comparing a provider against a composite unit projected onto a frontier.

DEA offers many advantages when applied to the problem of quality measurement. First, the models are non-parametric and do not require a prescribed functional form (Charnes et al. 1994). Second, unlike statistical regression which averages performance across many service providers, DEA estimates best practice by evaluating the performance behavior of each individual provider, pitting each provider against every other provider in the sample. The analysis identifies the amount of the performance deficiency and the source. Third, unlike regression and other statistical methods, DEA can handle multiple independent variables, so the analysis produces a single, overall measure of best results observed.

Finally, in order to identify those providers who achieved the best results, DEA groups providers into homogenous sub-groups. Providers that lie on the frontier achieved the best possible results and are rated 100%. Providers that behaved like those on the frontier, but do not lie on the surface under-performed, and their performance is measured by their distance from the frontier. Thus the analysis not only provides a measure of their relative performance, but also uncovers sub-groups of providers similar in their behavior or similar in the focus of their attention to performance.

Although the mathematical details and the computational aspects of optimal solutions are beyond the scope of this chapter, the following illustration explains how DEA works in estimating outcome frontiers. For an explanation of the DEA models used, see the appendix. Although DEA could be applied to any type of quality information, the following nursing home example is used to illustrate how to measure improvements in functional status and decision-making efficiency using DEA.

Theoretical Background: How DEA Works

To illustrate how DEA works, consider a group of 6 nursing homes each with 100 patients whose bed mobility, eating, and toilet use have been traced for a period of six months. Table 2 displays the overall functional status of the 100 patients in each of the six homes from quarter 1 to quarter 3. That situation can be depicted graphically in Figure 1 as a piecewise linear envelopment surface.

Change in Nursing home	Functional Status Q1	Functional Status Q3
N1	.15	.40
N2	.15	.14
N3	.35	.35
N4	.30	.15
N5	.40	.50
N6	.20	.30

Table 2. Nursing Home Outcomes: 100 Patients Traced for Six Months

In Figure 1, DEA floats a line in a 'northwesterly' direction to identify those nursing homes that had the greatest improvement in functional quality over the six-month period. Nursing homes N1 and N5 had the greatest improvement in the functional independence of their patient populations and the dotted lines connecting N1 and N5 represent the best practice frontier.

The vertical lines above N2, N6, N4, and N3 represents the potential improvements in quality outcomes if N2, N4, N6, and N3 had performed as well as N1 and N5. Note that since the initial functional status is a non-discretionary variable, the potential improvement can only occur along the vertical line. Associated with each under-performing nursing home is an optimal comparison point on the frontier that is a convex combination of the nursing homes. For example, N4 could be projected onto the best practice frontier at point X. The performance measure is the linear distance from the frontier expressed as a percent: 90%, 84% and so on. To be rated 100%, the nursing homes must be on the best practice surface.

In this simple two-dimensional example, the homes with the best improvements in functional status were identified. DEA is capable of assessing quality with dozens of indicators in n-dimensional space. For a more detailed explanation, see the appendix and for a complete mathematical explanation see Charnes et al. (1994).

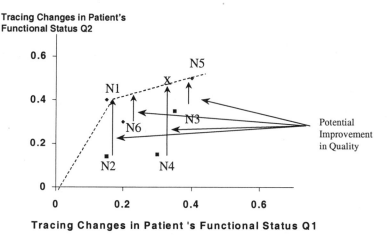

Chilingerian 1998

Figure 1. DEA Functional Frontier

Measuring Outcome and Efficiency Frontiers: An Application

To illustrate the ideas discussed above, the DEA discussed in the appendix will be used to find a quality-outcome frontier and an efficient practices frontier of 476 nursing homes[6] in Massachusetts (United States) in 1993. The study file on decision-making efficiency and outcomes used in this illustration was taken from a larger data base collected for each of the 476 nursing homes by the Massachusetts Rate Setting Commission.

The inputs and outputs for the productive efficiency dimension are displayed in figure 2, and are, largely, self-explanatory. The nine resource inputs are full time equivalent (FTE) registered nurses, FTE licensed practical nurses, and FTE nurse aides, FTE other labor, and medical supplies and drugs, clinical and other supplies, and claimed fixed costs (a proxy for capital). Since DEA can handle incommensurate data, the FTEs are in quantities, and supplies and costs are measured in dollars. The outputs are the quantity of resident days broken into three payer groups: Medicare (a national program to pay for elderly care), Medicaid (a state program to pay for impoverished residents), and Private (largely self-paying residents).

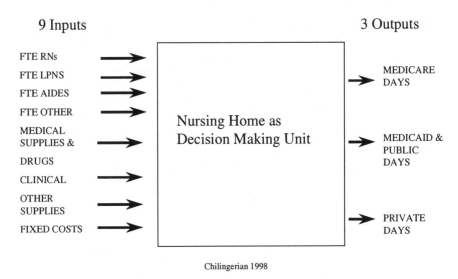

9 Inputs   3 Outputs

FTE RNs

FTE LPNS   MEDICARE
                                                                           DAYS
FTE AIDES

FTE OTHER

MEDICAL   Nursing Home as
SUPPLIES &   Decision Making Unit   MEDICAID &
                                                                           PUBLIC
DRUGS   DAYS

CLINICAL

OTHER
SUPPLIES
                                                                           PRIVATE
FIXED COSTS   DAYS

Chilingerian 1998

Figure 2. DEA Model Used to Measure Decision-Making Efficiency

Nursing home outcomes can be difficult to measure. Nursing homes in the United States, have several critical clinical indicators that are routinely monitored (Clark and Nottingham, 1997). These indicators are monitored with control charts to observe serious deviations from the mean. Among the typical clinical indicators such as facility infection rates, patient falls, weight loss , medication errors, number of pressure ulcers, are the change in activity of daily living (ADLs) conditions. When there are changes in two or more ADLs the number of patients improving and the number of patients with declines are tracked in US nursing homes (Clark and Nottingham, 1997).

Outcome measures for the nursing homes were developed from the Management Minutes Questionnaire (MMQ). This is the case-mix reimbursement tool used in several states in the United States and in particular is used in the state of Massachusetts to pay nursing homes for the services they provide to Medicaid residents. The MMQ collects information on the level of assistance that nursing home residents need from staff members to carry out activities of daily living such as dressing, eating, and moving about.

Fries (1990) explains that the MMQ index is constructed for each resident based on a spectrum of resident characteristics, each with a specified weight. Values are supposed to correspond to actual nursing times, so the total should correspond to total staffing needs for the resident. Weights are derived from expert opinion rather than statistical analysis, and total weights are adjusted with time values added for each of the items measured.

Changes in overall resident functioning (determined by measuring the change in MMQ scores over two quarters) were used as a proxy for quality of care. These variables depict the direction of functional status change (improvement, maintenance or decline) experienced by the residents during the last six months. Changes in a positive or static direction (improvement or maintenance) will be used as proxies for high quality care (controlling for health status) and changes in a negative direction (decline) will be used as a proxy for a decrease in the quality of care.

The proportion of residents who were independent in mobility and eating, and continent were traced for 6 months from quarter 1 to quarter 3. If we consider how a patient's functional status changes over time, whether a nursing home is improving, maintaining or declining, these changes become an outcome measurement tool. In particular, resident functional improvement was monitored by three activities of daily living: bed mobility, eating, and toilet use. The model used and the variables are displayed in Figure 3.

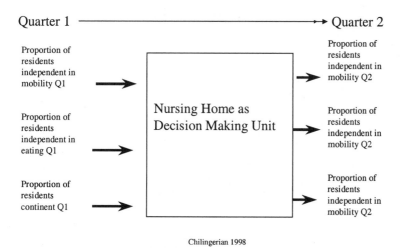

Chilingerian 1998

Figure 3. DEA Model Used to Measure Outcome Frontiers

Analysis of Preliminary Results

The DEA model identified 90 or 20% of the nursing homes on the best practice efficiency frontier and 41 or 9% of the nursing homes on the best practice quality frontier. The average decision-making efficiency score was 81%, which means that the potential reduction in the use of resources is 19%. The average quality score was 74%, which means that the functional status outcomes could potentially be improved by 26%.

The linear programming formulations estimate the savings in labor and other expenses. The potential savings in labor is 1,034 registered nurses out of 3,387, 1,204 licensed practical nurses out of 4,658, and 4,856 nurse aides out of 8,046. The potential savings in drugs, other medical supplies and material was $196,353,710 out of a total of $586,557,444 in expenses. These preliminary findings could be used to sharpen a second stage analysis of the factors associated with improved outcomes and efficient use of resources.

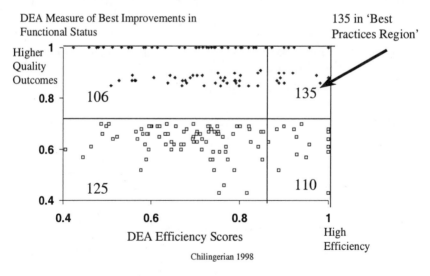

Figure 4. Two-Dimensional Summary DEA Measure of Change in Functional Status and Productive Efficiency

Figure 4 plots the DEA measure of the changes in functional status against a DEA measure of the decision-making efficiency for the 476 nursing homes in the data set. By partitioning this two-dimensional summary of nursing home performance at the means (81% and 74%), four categories of performers emerge: 135 with high quality outcome and high efficiency; 106 with high quality outcomes but lower efficiency; 110 with low quality outcomes but high efficiency; and 125 with lower quality outcomes and low efficiency. Each of these unique and exhaustive categories can be further analyzed to explore the factors associated with each category of performance. By studying the interaction of these two dimensions of performance, it may be possible to gain better insight into quality and efficiency.

Conclusions

This chapter has introduced another way of thinking about quality by addressing the problem of multi-dimensionality and using DEA to estimate one dimension of quality *outcomes*. The DEA methodology was extended to the problem of exploring outcome frontiers in nursing homes. The illustration opens the possibility of developing independent measures for each of the five dimensions of quality using frontier methods.

Two DEA models were used to assess the outcomes achieved by 476 nursing homes in 1993 and to compute productive efficiency scores. The results suggest a wide range of performance among the nursing homes. Only 135 nursing homes achieved better than a 74% outcome rating and a better than an 81% efficiency rating. The slack associated with the less efficient homes supports the hypothesis that a substantial amount could be saved, if every nursing home were as good as those on the frontiers. More importantly, it suggests that efficient, high quality care was achieved by 135 homes.

DEA directs attention to the frontiers of clinical practice rather than the central tendencies or "average practices." While statistical approaches explain average performance, DEA aims to explain who achieves the best results and why. The combination of statistical and DEA approaches may allow researchers to derive a more complete explanation of the factors associated with quality outcomes. Based on the preliminary results outlined above, this application promises to be a fruitful application of the DEA methodology to the problem of quality measurement.

There are two real tests of quality frontier models. The first is whether frontier studies can offer new insights into why some health care providers fail to attain the best possible outcomes? The second, more critical test, is whether these new insights can be translated into changes in practice? To restate what one physician stated so eloquently; "quality is not how well or how frequently medical service is given, but how closely the result approaches the fundamental objectives of prolonging life, relieving distress, restoring functions, and preventing disability."

The *outcome quality measures* derived in this study are relative to the best practices observed in the sample of 1993 Massachusetts' nursing homes studied in the United States, and not the best practices that might be observed in a more extensive sample over time. In the future, DEA methods could be applied in an international context in which quality outcome frontiers would identify global best practices. Studies of domestic outcomes benchmarked relative to global quality frontiers may teach us new lessons about the commitment, competence, and coordination of various systems of care.

Star Quality: Recapping the Five Dimensions

Recently, a physician with an MBA asked: "Is there the equivalent of a bottom line in health care?" The medical profession and the policy makers may enjoy debating this issue for a few more decades. Alternatively, we can enter the 21st century ready to measure quality in terms of the major features or dimensions of quality as shown in Figure 5.

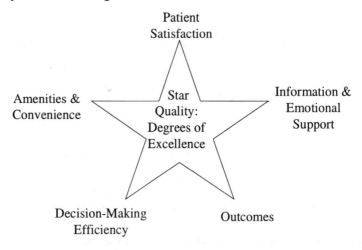

Figure 5: Five points of star quality

The two legs of "star quality" are outcomes and decision-making efficiency. At the apex, we see patient satisfaction, with emotional support/information and amenities/convenience at the flanks. Notwithstanding the difficulties of defining and measuring health care outputs, quality management can become a more tractable problem. Further progress depends on developing equitable report cards that considers quality in multi-dimensional configurations.

Although an argument was made that "star quality" is multi-dimensional, this paper focused on a single dimension—outcomes. Quality measures are available using statistical averages and new frontier approaches such as DEA. It is likely that frontier techniques such as DEA could be further extended to derive a single summary measure of relative quality when multiple dimensions (both quantitative and qualitative factors) are used. In pursuit of a balanced approach to quality measurement, future research should include all five dimensions. In every day parlance, quality medical care has a deeper meaning— it is understood as an overall "degree of excellence." Management control systems can work toward a goal of improving provider, caregivers, and delivery systems quality, if measurement systems benchmark excellence against the best care observed in practice and change provider behavior accordingly. Ultimately, management of quality has one fundamental goal—to benefit patients who need health care services, and expect high degrees of excellence.

Notes

I am very grateful to John Kimberly, Dianne Chilingerian, and Franz Schmidthaler for their encouragement and thoughtful comments. I also want to thank Mitchell Rabkin and Jerome Grossman who, perhaps inadvertently, suggested some of the dimensions underlying "star quality" to me. All views expressed and any mathematical errors are my responsibility.

[1] There is evidence of a very weak association between efficiency and quality, which suggests that they may best be thought of as independent dimensions (Chilingerian and Sherman 1990; Chilingerian 1994). Whether these features are unidimensional or multi-dimensional remains a research hypothesis that needs further empirical tests (Donabedian 1988).

[2] Recent research on service organization profitability suggests that the study of satisfaction must focus on the outliers—those who are *extremely* satisfied versus

extremely dissatisfied (Heskett et al. 1997). Merely 'satisfying' customers with services heads towards mediocrity and in the long run, is a formula for failure.

[3] Acceptable outcomes require expert judgments, a priori standards, or explicit expectations (Brook et al. 1996).

[4] Although there is some evidence that poor care processes do not necessarily lead to adverse outcomes, a compelling argument can be made that measures of the process of care are needed in quality assessment to avoid future negative outcomes (Crombie and Davies 1998). Since incorrect diagnoses, inappropriate treatments or poorly-administered treatments lead to excessive use of resources and clinical inefficiency, they are included under the decision making efficiency dimension.

[5] Although the frontier should be defined as the degree to which the observed performance a health care provider approaches its maximum potential, the maximum potential is a best-practice frontier based on the providers in the sample, and not all providers in the industry or that could conceivably exist.

[6] This study of 476 nursing homes excluded rest homes and nursing homes with incomplete data.

References

Ali, A. I., and L. M. Seiford. 1993. The Mathematical Programming Approach to Efficiency Analysis. In *The Measurement of Productive Efficiency*, edited by H. O. Fries, C.A. Knox Lovell, and S. S. Schmidt. New York: Oxford University Press.

Benner, P. 1984. *From Novice to Expert: Excellence and Power in Clinical Nursing Practice*. New York:Addison-Wesley Publishing Company.

Berwick, D. 1996. The Year of 'How:' New Systems for Delivering Health Care. *Quality Connections* 5 (1): 1-4

Blumenthal, D. 1996. Quality of Care: What Is It? *New England Journal of Medicine* 335(12):891-4.

Bodenheimer, T. 1999. The Movement for Improved Quality in Health Care. *New England Journal of Medicine* 340: 488-92.

Brook, R. H., E. A. McGlynn, and P. D. Cleary. 1996. Measuring Quality of Care. *New England Journal of Medicine* 335 (13): 966-9.

Charnes, A., W. Cooper, and E. Rhodes. 1978. Measuring the Efficiency of Decision Making Units. *European Journal of Operational Research* 2 (6): 429-44.

Charnes, A., W. Cooper, A. Y. Lewine, and L. M. Seiford. 1994. Basic DEA Models. In *Data Envelopment Analysis: Theory, Methodology, and Application*, edited by A. Charnes, W. Cooper, A. Y. Lewin, and L. M. Seiford. Boston, Massachusetts: Kluwer Academic Publishers.

Charnes, A., W. Cooper, B. Golany, L. Seiford, and J. Stutz. 1985. Foundations of Data Envelopment Analysis for Pareto-Koopmans Efficient Empirical Production Functions. *Journal of Econometrics* 30 (12): 91-107.

Chassin, M. R., and R. W.Galvin. 1998. The Urgent Need to Improve Health Care Quality. *Journal of the American Medical Association* 280:1000-1005.

Chilingerian, J. 1992. New Directions for Hospital Strategic Management: The Market for Efficient Care. *Health Care Management Review* 17 (4):73-80.

Chilingerian, J. 1994. Exploring Why Some Physicians' Hospital Practices Are More Efficient: Taking DEA Inside the Hospital. In *Data Envelopment Analysis: Theory, Methodology, and Application*, edited by A. Charnes, W. Cooper, A. Y. Lewin, and L. M. Seiford. Boston, Massachusetts: Kluwer Academic Publishers..

Chilingerian, J. 1995. Evaluating Physician Efficiency in Hospitals: A Multi-Variate Analysis of Best Practices. *European Journal of Operational Research* 80:548-74.

Chilingerian, J., and D. H. Sherman. 1990. Managing Physician Efficiency and Effectiveness in Providing Hospital Services. *Health Services Management Research* 3(1):3-15.

Clark, K. L., and A. Nottingham. 1997. Improving Quality in Integrated Health Care Systems. In *Improving Quality: A Guide to Effective Programs*, edited by I.N. Meisenheimer and G. Claire. Gaithersburg, Maryland: Aspen Publications.

Cohan, M. E., and S. M. Mareno. 1992. Improving Quality in Long-Term Care. In *Total Quality Management: The Health Care Pioneers*, edited by I. N.Meisenheimer and G. Claire. Chicago: American Hospital Association Publications.

Crombie, I. K., and H .T. O. Davies. 1998. Beyond Health Outcomes: The Advantages of Measuring Process. *Journal of Evaluation in Clinical Practice.* 4 (1): 31-8.

Davies, H. T. O. 1997. What's a Health Outcome? *Health Service Journal* 10: 22-3.

Davies, H.,T. O., and L. K. Crombie. 1997. Interpreting Health Outcomes. *Journal of Evaluation in Clinical Practice* 3 (3): 187-99.

Delbanco, T. L. 1992. Enriching the Doctor-Patient Relationship by Inviting the Patient's Perspective. *Annals of Internal Medicine* 116 (5): 414-18.

Donabedian, A. 1988. The Quality of Care: How Can It Be Assessed. *Journal of the American Medical Association* 260 (12):1743-48.

Eisenberg, J. M. 1986. *Doctors' Decisions and the Cost of Medical Care*. Ann Arbor, Michigan: Health Administration Press.

Ellwood, P. M. 1988. Outcomes Management. A Technology of Patient Experience. *New England Journal of Medicine* 318:1549-56.

Fries, B. E. 1990. Comparing Case-Mix Systems for Nursing Home Payment. *Health Care Financing Review* 11:103-14.

Glavin, M. P. V., and J. A. Chilingerian. 1998. Hospital Production and Medical Errors: Organizational Responses to Improve Care. *Current Topics in Management* 3:193-215.

Gold, M., and J. Wooldridge. 1995. Surveying Customer Satisfaction to Assess Managed Care Quality: Current Practices. *Health Care Financing Review* 16 (4):155-73.

Gumbel, E.J. 1958. *Statistics of Extremes*. New York: Columbia University Press.

Hemenway, D. 1984. *Prices and Choices: Microeconomic Vignettes*. Cambridge, Massachusetts: Ballinger Publishing Company.

Harris, J. E. The Internal Organization of Hospitals: Some Economic Implications. *The Bell Journal of Economics* 77: 467-82.

Herzlinger, R. 1997. *Market-Driven Care: Who Wins, Who Loses in the Transformation of America's Largest Service Industry*. Reading, Massachusetts: Addison-Wesley.

Heskett, J. L. 1986. *Managing in the Service Economy*. Boston: Harvard Business School Press.

Heskett, J. L., W. E. Sasser, and L. A. Schlesinger. 1997. *The Service Profit Chain*. New York: The Free Press.

Kenagy, J. W., D. M. Berwick, and M.F. Shore. 1999. Service Quality in Health Care. *Journal of the American Medical Association* 281 (7):661-5.

Levitan, S. E. 1992. *Providing Emotional Support*. Picker/Commonwealth Report 1(3). Boston: Beth Israel Hospital.

Lewin, A. Y., and J. W. Minton. 1986. Determining Organizational Effectiveness: Another Look and an Agenda for Research. *Management Science* 32 (5):514-38.

Meisenheimer, C. G. 1997. *Improving Quality: A Guide to Effective Programs*. Second edition. Gaithersburg, Maryland: Aspen Publications.

Melum, M. M. and M. K. Sinioris. 1992. *Total Quality Management: The Health Care Pioneers*. Chicago: American Hospital Association Publications.

de Pouvourville, G. 1997. Quality of Care Initiatives in the French Context. *International Journal for Quality in Health Care* 9 (3):163-70.

Schauffler, H. H., T. Rodriguez, and A. Milstein. 1996. Health Education and Patient Satisfaction. *The Journal of Family Practice* 42 (1):62-8.

Struebing, L. 1996. Customer Loyalty: Playing for Keeps. *Quality Progress*, 28 (2): 25-30.

Steffen, G. E. 1988. Quality Medical Care: A Definition. *Journal of the American Medical Association* 260(1):56-61.

Steffen, T.M., and P. C. Nystrom. 1997. Organizational Determinants of Service Quality in Nursing Homes. *Hospital and Health Services Administration* 42 (2): 179-91.

Appendix

DEA is linear programming based and requires solving a mathematical model that finds an optimal value for each health care provider. The optimal value is a performance rating that measures the distance of any provider from the frontier. Whereas regression proceeds with a single optimization, DEA proceeds with a series of optimizations—one for each provider unit. The availability of computer programs is extensive, and DEA is available even on spreadsheet packages such as Excel. The DEA package used in this chapter is called IDEAS, developed by Agha Iqbal Ali and available from 1 Consulting, PO Box 2453, Amherst MA, 01004, USA. The notation used here follows Charnes et al. 1994.

There are a variety of DEA models, each one determines an envelopment surface referred to as a "best practices" frontier. Two of these models will be discussed below: one for evaluating outcomes and another for evaluating decision-making efficiency.

A DEA model for outcome frontiers

The model that can be used to introduce an outcome-quality frontier is called the additive model (Charnes et al. 1985). The additive model is based on the idea of subtracting the functional status of the patient at the outset from the status attained after the care process. The resulting measure is expressed as a change in functional status based on the functional status achieved during Time Two (F_{T2}) minus (the functional status at the outset (F_{T1}). The numerical differences from F_{T1} to F_{T2} can be interpreted as improvements, deteriorations, or no change in outcomes.

The optimal value w^*_o is a rating that measures the distance that a particular nursing home being rated lies from the frontier. A separate linear programming model is run for each nursing home (or unit) whose outcomes are to be assessed. The additive model is shown below:

$$\max_{u, v, u_O} \quad w_o = u^T Y_o - v^T X_o + u_o$$

$$\text{s.t.} \quad u^T Y - v^T X + u_o 1 \leq 0$$

$$-u^T \leq -1$$

$$-v^T \leq -1$$

Additive model

Y represents the observed functional status variables at F_{T2} and X represents the initial functional status variables observed at F_{T1}. The additive model subtracts the functional status variable at F_{T2} from those at F_{T1}. The variables, u^T *and* v^T are the weights assigned by the linear program so $u^T Y$ is the weighted functional status at F_{T2} and $v^T X$ is the weighted functional status at F_{T1}. The model is constrained so that every nursing home is included in the optimization such that the range of scores will be between 0 and 100%. [1] The u^T and v^T are constrained to be non-negative.

For the problem of developing a frontier measure of improvements or deterioration in functional status, the additive has a number of advantages (see Charnes et al. 1994). The model does not focus on a proportional reduction of inputs or an augmentation of outputs. It offers a global measure of a distance from a frontier, by giving an equal focus on functional status before and after by maximizing the functional improvement between time periods (characterized as the difference between T_1 and T_2). Another advantage of the additive model is that it is translation invariant, which means we can add a vector to the inputs and outputs and although we get a new data set, the estimates of best practice and the outcome measures will be the same. This model will be applied to a nursing home data set to find a DEA outcome frontier and a DEA decision-making efficiency frontier.

A DEA Model for efficiency frontiers
To locate best practices from an efficiency standpoint, an input-oriented model with constant returns to scale is often selected (Charnes et al. 1994). This model measures overall technical and scale efficiency. The model, shown below answers the following question: Given the quantity of residents or patients) cared for, could the inputs be reduced? This approach can be used not only to monitor variations in the utilization of resources and identify which clinical inputs might be reduced, but also to help researchers understand why medical practices vary (Chilingerian 1994).

---

[1] A DEA model can be formulated to accommodate the fact that the functional status variables at FT1 are non-discretionary.

$$\max_{u,v} \quad w_o = u^T Y_o$$

$$\text{s.t.} \quad v^T X_o = 1$$

$$u^T Y \_ v^T X \leq 0$$

$$\rightarrow$$

$$-u^T \leq -\varepsilon 1$$

$$\rightarrow$$

$$-v^T \leq -\varepsilon 1$$

Input—Oriented CCR Model

The model used to evaluate efficiency is expressed as a ratio of weighted outputs divided by weighted inputs: $u^T Y / v^T X$. By setting the denominator, $v^T X$ equal to 1 and maximizing the weighted outputs, $u^T Y$, this model can be solved as a linear program. Every nursing home is evaluated separately and given the best possible efficiency score in a range between 0 and 100%. The u^T and v^T are constrained to be a non-negative number and less than or equal to a very small (non-archimedean) number.

Chapter 9

Rethinking Quality: Complexity and Context in Health Care

Leonard B. Lerer

Health care has been a fertile and lucrative area for quality management and its practitioners. Quality improvement methods are increasingly being used in areas such as primary health care (Fischer, Solberg and Kottke 1998), mental health (Sluyter 1998), and by publicly funded agencies, such as Medicaid and the US Veterans Affairs Health Services (Landon, Tobias and Epstein 1998; Young, Charns and Barbour 1997). Countries with national health insurance, such as the United Kingdom, have vigorously espoused quality improvement (see Thomson 1998) and even in nations as diverse as Russia, Brazil and South Africa, quality measurement and improvement methodologies are being increasingly implemented[1]. Quality, now used as a marketing attribute by private health providers, has become part of the daily discourse of health.

Total quality management (TQM) or continuous quality improvement (CQI) within the health sector has been extensively reviewed and discussed (Blumenthal 1996a; Carman et al 1996). The Institute of Medicine defines quality of care as "the degree to which health services for individuals and populations increase the likelihood of desired health outcomes and are consistent with current knowledge" (Chassin, Galvin and The National Roundtable on Health Care Quality 1998). This definition, first proposed in the early 1990's, indicates the breadth of the quality concept within the health sector and an orientation towards health outcomes and their measurement.

There are many reasons for the enthusiastic reception and integration of industrial, and to an extent, service quality approaches within health institutions. De Pouvourville (1997) attributes an increase in interest in quality issues to pressures from financial stakeholders for more cost-effective and transparent health service provision. This observation appears to be valid in most industrialized countries, as cost constraints often force organizational change (Tonneau 1997). Perhaps the most important driver of quality has been managed health care (MHC) and while it is not my purpose to discuss the relationship between quality and MHC, it is important to note that most definitions of MHC stress quality as one of its goals. If one goes further and includes the application of standardized business practices as a component of MHC, then the role of quality, especially at an operational or process level becomes even more apparent.

The science of quality and its management have become integral parts of industrialized country health systems. In broadly attributing the "process focus" of quality management within the health sector to its origins in the manufacturing sector, I first raise the possibility that it may not take some of the unique attributes of health care[2] into account, and then go on to discuss the limitations of current "off the shelf" quality management approaches in dealing with the range of stakeholders and institutional complexity. The chapter ends with a proposal for a more "context"—based or clinical model of quality that prioritizes the patient or health care consumer and accommodates the complexity of health care institutions.

The Techniques of Quality

A terminological cornucopia with words and phrase such as CQI, TQM, quality assurance (QA), CQI teams, performance measures, benchmarking, accreditation and quality action programs is a feature of quality in health care. These terms represent the methodology, tools or as I prefer, techniques[3] whereby quality is practiced in the health sector. Quality measurement systems and management methods have demonstrated utility in clinical practice (Chassin 1996) and audit improves the practice of healthcare professionals, especially in areas such as diagnostic test selection and drug prescribing. At a clinical level, performance measurement for all aspects of care is regarded as the main route to quality improvement (Palmer 1997). However, as recent reviews by Thomson et al. (1998a,b) indicate, measurement or audit alone may not be the most effective approach to change professional behavior, and the biomedical literature provides little advice as to complementary approaches to quality improvement.

The range of perspectives on quality in health care is largely determined by the interests of stakeholders (Donabedian 1988) and a patient's concept of a good quality health encounter (usually an interaction with a sympathetic caregiver), often differs from that of a health care manager, who may look only at cost and outcome criteria. For managers, the quality focus has been on outcomes measurement, as the only available response to utilization and quality-based reimbursement incentives. The substrate upon which quality intervention is practiced varies considerably between country and institution. While the lines of "fracture" between curative care, managerial and community functions may be reasonably clear in a large acute care hospital[4], industrialized country health systems are moving towards institutional arrangements in which financial, administrative and social responsibilities are shared among medical staff, communities and administrators. In this environment, power-relations become increasingly important, as key groups adjust to new demands and opportunities. Young (1997) describes this from an "ideological perspective" noting that it is relatively easy for health professionals to adjust to an overriding market/consumer ideology, while managers often have to use audits and other "technologies" to exert their power over physicians.

Although quality in health care may be difficult to define, the settings in which it is applied and many of the methods used, are easy to identify. Good quality care is appropriate, effective and accessible and conforms to some measure of efficiency or cost-effectiveness. Private and public health systems emphasize different parts of the quality spectrum, but most elements of health care quality can be defined by their role in the process of care. With this in mind, I propose that current approaches to quality be best divided into three groups; access, care and outcome[5].

Access Quality

This incorporates all aspects governing the accessibility of care to the patient. As access quality also includes elements of social justice (mainly barriers to obtaining care), it has not been stressed by private health care providers. Access has become of increasing importance, in the context of screening and disease management for chronic conditions, where insurers have found that early interventions may result in long-term savings. Another access consideration relates to the over- and misuse of health services and procedures[6] and the dangerous consequences of the proliferation of medical procedures (Fisher and Welch 1999).

Quality of Care

This includes a range of existing quality parameters in all areas of health services including prevention, resources for diagnosis and treatment, facility quality and the speed with which clinical decisions are made. Most aspects of the encounter between patients, physicians and nurses fall in the quality of care category and much of the quality improvement literature focuses on this area. The quality of services, especially from nursing staff, physicians and staff responsible for hospital logistics are coming under increasing scrutiny.

Outcome Quality

In its recent consensus document, the Institute of Medicine (see Chassin, Galvin and The National Roundtable on Health Care Quality 1998), stressed the advances in the measurement of quality in American health care and the need for further dissemination of best-practices, especially those based on randomized controlled trials and systematic reviews. Most of such measurement is based on patient outcomes, which are also used for benchmarking and institutional comparisons. The measurements include morbidity and mortality, health and functional status and quality of life, patient satisfaction, hospital operational performance and supplier quality.

Process	Quality measurement	Example
Access	Per-capita use of preventive, diagnostic and curative facilities Pharmaceutical consumption	Measurement of the population-adjusted distribution of technology, procedures and facilities
Care	Data on procedures, patient satisfaction, expenditures, costs, savings Quality scorecards	IT-based management protocols
Outcome	Morbidity, mortality and quality of life data Financial data	Risk-adjusted comparisons

Table 1: Process Quality in Health Care

Table 1 highlights some aspects of process quality; this list is however far from comprehensive and some practical examples exist, representing best practices in this area (see Shulkin 1997; Shulkin and Joshi 1999; Chilingerian 1999).

Limitations of Quality Interventions

There is a growing body of knowledge, as with any maturing management approach, about pitfalls in the implementation of health care quality (Shortell et al. 1995; Chase and Carr-Hill 1994). TQM, in managed care settings, has largely focused on cost-containment and standardization of procedures. This approach aims to produce short-term, quantifiable results (McLaughlin and Kaluzny 1997) and is, as I also argue, largely process-oriented. When quality improvement is prioritized in a health service, a danger exists that its key elements will be punitive audits and intensification of managerial control (Thomson 1998). Physician skepticism about quality has been partially justified by failed and often foolish quality improvement initiatives and the almost inevitable association between quality management and financial constraints (Chassin 1996). Similarly, claims that TQM can substantially improve hospital performance and competitiveness and result in a sustained improvement in quality of care, have been exaggerated (Bigelow and Arndt 1995; Blumenthal and Epstein 1996). While a number of hospital groups provide superb examples of the successful application of elements of quality management (see Shulkin 1997; Fontaine et al. 1997), no health system can in its entirety, be put forward as a gold-standard.

The Limits of Quality
Observations of hastily implemented and inappropriate "off-the-shelf" quality interventions in health care, while highlighting the inappropriate application of quality tools, also raise a more fundamental question; whether quality management is the most appropriate approach to improving the core business of the health sector—patient care? The sustainability of health care QI initiatives based on audit and control has been questioned (Thomson and Barton 1994), as have industrial quality management techniques such as error reduction or Six Sigma quality (Chassin 1998). A more profound difference between

industrial and health care quality is highlighted by a key tenet of the industrial process oriented philosophy described by Chung (1999:188) as; "if one takes care of the process, the product will take care of itself". The link between process and product is much clearer in manufacturing than in health care. No matter how good their systems, physicians, hospital managers and MHC providers are forced to deal with individual patients who respond differently to standardized intervention protocols and whose autonomy must be respected, even if they make ostensibly unwise health-related choices.

The limitations of quantitative approaches to quality are also rooted in the fact that patients, and increasingly health care purchasers such as large employers have different benchmarks against which they compare the quality of service providers. From the perspective of a consumer, many quantitative performance measures may be of limited relevance and may tell little about the quality of the interaction, at an individual level, between the patient and health care organization (Galvin 1998). While innovations such as evidence-based medicine are grounded in conformance with clinical criteria and quantitative quality measurement (Drummond 1998), it remains to be seen whether this will be sufficient to satisfy the needs of all health care consumers for overarching indicators of quality.

Complexity

Quality in health care, as described by management theorists and practiced by managers and consultants, has been criticized as not having an adequate philosophical foundation and not being cognizant of the political, economic and social milieu in which healthcare exists (Loughlin 1996). The largely quantitative criteria for judging quality limit our understanding of the true nature of quality in the complex health care environment. Advances in technology and disease management have challenged our current concept of the hospital (Kimberly 1998), and quality is increasingly being considered in settings such as community-based care and telemedicine (Shortell, Gillies and Devers 1995). The increasing sophistication of treatment, technological complexity, the magnitude of data on best practices and better informed patients are driving integration of processes within health care (Blumenthal 1996b).

We are, however, beginning to know more about the complexity of health care institutions, the often conflicting agendas of stakeholders, the challenge of diversity and variability of processes (Minvielle 1997; Tonneau 1997,1999).

Decision-making and control in hospitals is often not based on a simple model of hierarchical control and it is thus difficult to institute "classical" TQM methodologies (Arndt and Bigelow 1995; Kennedy 1998). Suffice it to observe that many quality assurance approaches do not cope well with resource constraints, institutional power-relations and ethical challenges[7]. Medical professionals often judge quality interventions too prematurely and harshly, failing to accept that quality management is in itself an evolutionary process. Some physicians claim that just as they become comfortable with quality audit, peer review and accreditation procedures (and perhaps have a better understanding of how to manipulate them for their own ends), they are forced to become involved in new initiatives to transform their organizations. Hospital administrators facing an almost perpetual "crisis of control" resort to TQM as an intervention against cost and other pressures, regardless of the long-term consequences or the lack of stakeholder buy-in (Glouberman and Mintzberg 1998a). Hospital administrators, nurses and doctors often identify different "quality-issues" as being of importance (Sales et al. 1995) and at worst, quality becomes a weapon on the ideological battleground between managers and health professionals (Young 1997)[8].

Another aspect of complexity is related to the variability in health outcomes among patients receiving the same intervention or treatment. It is important to carefully examine the discourse of quality measurement, to ensure that it is appropriate in an environment of biomedical "uncertainty". Variability of outcome is enmeshed in our perception and faith in the medical profession, but remains relatively unexplored in the quality arena[9].

Rethinking Quality

I have already alluded to quality in health care, as being something more than simply an aggregation of methods, tools and techniques—best defined as *process*. This viewpoint is certainly not original, as Enthoven and Vorhaus (1997) for example, have articulated a vision of quality in health, which includes excellence in quality improvement, physician attitudes, patient involvement and financing. The position that quality has become almost exclusively process focussed can be criticized as not reflecting the range of efforts to improve services and better train personnel, being undertaken under the quality in health care banner. The main feature of the health quality movement, especially in the USA, has however been quantitative measurement of processes, especially outcomes. Proposals to improve quality within the health sector almost invariably include rigorous measurement, standardization, evidence based protocols and increased used of IT[10]. Health care, however, is both a precise and imprecise science, deeply intertwined with social and ethical issues and similarly, health care management shares these inherent features[11]. As the health sector faces the challenge of integrating quality management across the entire spectrum of care (Shulkin 1997), it is not sufficient to merely be followers, exclusively using existing quality tools designed mainly for manufacturing and specific services. The management literature has for some time recognized the limitations of using a directive, results oriented strategic approach (see Alvesson and Wilmott 1996) and many industries have undertaken the transformation of the quality paradigm, from that of conformity and control to the creation of an customer-oriented, integrated and continuously learning and improving organization[12]. Although it may be appropriate for the health sector to follow innovations in industrial quality management, these techniques cannot simply be imported and incorporated in an unchanged state. If health care remains simply a follower, then it risks further disenchantment with its quality initiatives.

Health care specific models that make quality implicit rather than enforced are required. This concept should not be regarded as alien, as some implicit aspects of quality can be identified in health service delivery (Tonneau 1999). Charns and Young's (1999) use of the terms *programming coordination* (procedures and protocols) and *feedback coordination* (inter-personal interaction) goes some way towards highlighting what I see as the primary and two interacting components of quality in health care; *process* and *context*. Process has been described earlier in this chapter as comprised of access, care and outcomes (see Table 1). Context can be regarded as the broader milieu or environment in which process quality exists. Rather than proposing a radical revision or complex model of quality in health care, the "rethinking" of quality should focus on two core components of context; the *patient or consumer* and the *organization*.

Patient/Consumer Context

Current health care QI methods, although certainly considering patient satisfaction and aspects of service, mainly measure post-hoc outcomes.

Although some "lip-service" is paid to the patient, whatever power individual health care consumers had, has been decreased by managed care and new structures for the delivery of care. The failure to recognize that the business of health care is the improvement of health status at an individual level inevitably leads conditions under which quality initiatives cannot succeed. Sustainable QI in health care, as in service operations management, needs to refocus on core components such as patient or consumer oriented performance measurement, operations improvement, customer service and technology development (see Johnston 1999).

Organizational Context

TQM has been based on rapidly teaching organizations various best practices, rather than on nurturing learning and leveraging the diverse knowledge and skills found in most healthcare settings (McLaughlin and Kaluzny 1997). It is outside the scope of this chapter to explore the relationship between quality, learning and knowledge within organizations (see Wilson and Asay 1999); suffice it to observe that knowledge-based organizations have the capacity to innovate, derive strategic advantage, and respond to customer needs (Nonaka 1991; Nonaka and Konno 1998). There is a growing interest in the concepts of knowledge and learning within the health sector. Pharmaceutical companies are, for example, taking the lead in using "intellectual capital" to ensure that innovative thinking is sustained, especially in drug development. The nurturing of knowledge and skills goes hand in hand with the recognition of the complexity of health care organizations. As discussed earlier, one of the major problems with the available quality management armamentarium lies not so much in the methods, but rather in the fact that quality interventions are often "overlaid" onto complex organizations.

The Case for Context Quality

The process/context concept can be criticized as not recognizing that many of the elements described as context are indeed dealt with in TQM programs. Human resource development, intra-organizational communication, service improvement and exercises to recognize institutional barriers to QI are certainly part of current quality initiatives. However, forcing a distinction between process and context facilitates the recognition that far more resources need to be devoted to the qualitative or softer issues in the quality arena. It may be possible to modify existing quality management methods to ensure that they are more cognizant of complexity, organizational and consumer issues. The distinction between process and context also assists in driving quality improvement, as it to some extent compensates for the lack of quality drivers, such as inter-firm rivalry and the demand for innovation, which are not often not present in health care settings.

Translating a broader model of quality in health care into action does not require radical modification of current quality management tools, but rather extensive reflection among all stakeholders as to the nature of the health care customer and the organizational structure that will best nurture knowledge sharing and teamwork. Coordination (Charns and Young 1999) and implicit quality (Tonneau 1999) in health care organizations may be proxies for context, but further research is required to refine the concept of context quality. The use of futures or scenarios can also be considered as this often evokes consideration of organizational transformation and the new health care consumer. Hospitals may question the value of exercises that focus on institutional issues, claiming that their structure and control are determined externally, by administrative boards, health insurers, governments or regional authorities. However, potential avenues for reform, entrepreneurship and innovation exist in even the most rules-bound organizations (Mintzberg 1996; Glouberman and Mintzberg 1998b).

Conclusions

Broadening the concept of quality within the health sector is not without attendant dangers. Kimberly (1997) alerts us to the potential barriers to introducing a widespread quality consultation in health, particularly the divisions between the various stakeholders. The power of particular groups such as professional organizations, public servants and politicians rapidly manifests when quality is perceived as a threat. If, however, quality is not to be relegated to the ranks of another passing management fad or fashion, it must extend beyond operations or process and into the very context of health care, the customer or patient and the organization. Industrial quality techniques have changed the way that modern health care is delivered and benchmarked, and the next challenge lies not so much in the refinement of quality methods, but rather in the search for ways to extend quality management beyond purely process issues.

The legacy of quality in health care is firmly grounded in the ethical tenets of non-malfeasance and beneficence (Beauchamp and Childress 1989); however financial and administrative procedures make it difficult to consider the primacy of the patient (or health care consumer). Moving beyond process into context quality requires consideration of the very purpose or core business of health care and provides the opportunity to rethink quality in the health sector.

Notes

[1] See various authors in the May 1998 Issue of the Joint Commission on Quality Improvement Journal (Volume 24, No 5).

[2] For a detailed discussion on the differences of the health care industry, see Walston, Kimberly and Burns (1996) and the various references they cite.

[3] The term *technique* is used more to describe a *technique of power* than simply a methodology. Whilst I do not explore this in any depth, my argument relates to the way that quality is used to exert overt and covert influence within organizations in a Foucaultian sense (Dreyfuss and Rabinow 1982).

[4] For a detailed discussion , see Glouberman and Mintzberg 1998a, 1998b. The authors largely attribute the complexity in managing acute care hospitals to the differentiation between curative, care, administrative and community components.

[5] This classification is, to a limited extent, similar to Donabedian's (1989) use of *structure, process* and *outcome*. The classification replaces structure with access, as I argue that structure is a component of organizational context rather than part of the quality process. Process is used as a more general term to cover access, care and outcome.

[6] The Institute of Medicine (IOM) has recently produced a Consensus Statement on the need to improve quality in health care (see Chassin, Galvin and The National Roundtable on Quality in Health Care 1998). This Consensus Panel classifies "quality problems" as due to underuse (the failure to provide a health service that would result in a favorable outcome), overuse (providing a health service whose potential for harm exceeds its beneficial purposes) and misuse (preventable complications from an appropriate service). For a detailed example of strategies that "ration" access to unnecessary procedures, see Chassin (1996).

[7] For example, the use of clinical guidelines, reviewed by Huttin (1997), is hampered by the complexity of medical "systems" making results of this intervention sub-optimal.

[8] Young (1997) also identifies the role of the clinical audit as a strategic weapon in the hands of administrators seeking to exert control over physicians. Although the examples used are from the United Kingdom, her comments resonate clearly with experiences in managed care in the USA, where some payers have used clinical guidelines and best-practices as a cost-containment method.

[9] I am grateful to John Kimberly for alerting me to the "differential contexts" of health care quality.

[10]Eddy (1998:17) makes an eloquent case for performance measurement. On process measures, he writes that: "Unlike many of their companion health outcomes, processes tend to be frequent, immediate, controllable and rarely confounded by other factors."

[11]Chilingerian (1999) discusses the evidence supporting a "multi-dimensional" concept of quality.

[12]Cole (1998) provides a history of the transformation of the "quality movement". Of particular interest is the role of the USA as a follower of Japanese trends in quality management. One can contend that health care is largely a follower of industry in the quality arena.

References

Alvesson, M., and H. Wilmott. 1996. *Making sense of management: a critical introduction*. New York:Sage Books.

Arndt, M., Bigelow B. 1995. The implementation of total quality management in hospitals: how good is the fit? Health Care Management Review 20(4): 7-14.

Beauchamp, T. L., and J. F. Childress. 1989. *Principles of Bioethics*. New York: Oxford University Press.

Bigelow, B., and M. Arndt. 1995. Total quality management: field of dreams? *Health Care Management Review* 20(4): 15-25.

Blumenthal, D. 1996a. Quality of care—what is it? *New England Journal of Medicine* 335: 891-94.

Blumenthal, D. 1996b. The origins of the quality-of-care debate. *New England Journal of Medicine* 335:1146-49.

Blumenthal, D., and A. M. Epstein. 1996. The role of physicians in the future of quality management. *New England Journal of Medicine* 335: 1328-31.

Carman, J. M., S. M. Shortell, and R. W. Foster. 1996. Keys for the successful implementation of total quality management in hospitals. *Health Care Management Review* 21: 48-60.

Charns, M. P., and G. J. Young. 1999. Coordination and patient outcomes. In *The Quality Imperative,* edited by J. R. Kimberly and E. Minvielle. London:Imperial College Press.

Chassin, M. R. 1996. Improving the quality of care. *New England Journal of Medicine* 335: 1060-63.

Chase, E., and R. Carr-Hill. 1994. The dangers of managerial perversion: quality assurance in primary care. *Health Policy and Planning* 9: 267-78.

Chassin, M. R., R. W. Galvin and The National Roundtable on Health Care Quality. 1998. The urgent need to improve health care quality: Institute of Medicine Roundtable on Health Care Quality. *Journal of the American Medical Association* 280: 1000-5.

Chassin, M. R. 1998. Is health care ready for Six Sigma quality? *Milbank Quarterly* 76(4): 565-91.

Chassin M. R. 1996. Quality improvement nearing the 21st century: prospects and perils. *American Journal of Medical Quality* 11(1): S4-7.

Chilingerian, J. 1999. Evaluating quality outcomes against best practice: A new frontier. In *The Quality Imperative,* edited by J. R. Kimberly and E. Minvielle. London:Imperial College Press.

Chung, C. H. 1999. It is the process: A philosophical foundation for quality management. *Total Quality Management* 10(2): 187-97.

Cole, R. E. 1998. Learning from the quality movement: What did and didn't happen and why. *California Management Review* 41(1): 43-73.

Donabedian, A. 1966. Evaluating the quality of medical care. *Milbank Memorial Fund Quarterly* 44: 167-206.

Donabedian, A. 1988. The quality of care: how can it be assessed? *Journal of the American Medical Association* 260: 1743-48.

Donabedian, A. 1989. Institutional and professional responsibilities in quality assurance. *Quality Assurance in Health Care* 1(1): 3-11.

Drummond, M. 1998. Evidence-based medicine and cost-effectiveness: uneasy bedfellows. *American College of Physicians Journal Club* 3: 133-34.

Fischer, L. R., L. I. Solberg, and T. Kottke. 1998. Quality improvement in primary care clinics. *Joint Commission Journal on Quality Improvement* 24(7): 361-70.

Dreyfus, H. L., and P. Rabinow. 1982. *Michel Foucault: Beyond structuralism and hermeneutics.* New York: Harvester and Wheatsheaf.

Durand-Zaleski, I. and P. Durieux. 1999. The development of evaluation units in French hospitals: experiences and limitations. In *The Quality Imperative,* edited by J. R. Kimberly and E. Minvielle. London: Imperial College Press.

Eddy, D. M. 1998. Performance measurement: problems and solutions. *Health Affairs* 17(4): 7-25.

Enthoven, A. C., and C. B. Vorhaus. 1997. A vision of quality in health care delivery. *Health Affairs* 16(4): 44-57.

Fisher, E. S., and H. G. Welch. 1999. Avoiding the unintended consequences of the growth in medical care. *Journal of the American Medical Association* 281: 446-53.

Fontaine, A., P. Vinceneux, A. P. Puchet Traversat, and C. Catala. 1997. Toward quality improvement in a French hospital: Structures and culture. *International Journal for Quality in Health Care* 9 (3): 177-81.

Galvin, R. S. 1998. Are performance measures relevant? *Health Affairs* 17(4): 29-31.

Gillies, R. K., S. E. Reynolds, S. M. Shortell, E. F. X. Hughes, P. J. Budetti, A. W. Rademaker, C. Hang, and D. S. Dranove. 1999. The barriers and facilitators for implementing continuous quality improvement. In *The Quality Imperative*, edited by J. R. Kimberly and E. Minvielle. London: Imperial College Press.

Glouberman, R. S., and H. Mintzberg. 1998a. *Managing the care of health and the cure of disease, Part 1: Differentiation.* INSEAD Working Paper 98/49/SM. Fontainebleau, France: INSEAD.

Glouberman, R. S., and H. Mintzberg. 1998b. *Managing the care of health and the cure of disease, Part 2: Integration.* INSEAD Working Paper 98/49/SM. Fontainebleau, France: INSEAD.

Huttin, C. 1997. The use of clinical guidelines to improve medical practice: Main issues in the United States. *International Journal for Quality in Health Care* 9 (3): 207-14.

Johnston, R. 1999. Service operations management: return to roots. *International Journal of Operations and Production Management* 19(2): 104-24.

Kennedy, M. P. 1998. Implementation of quality improvement methodology and the health care profession. *Journal of Quality in Clinical Practice* 18(2): 143-50.

Kimberly, J. R. 1997. Assessing quality in health care: Issues in measurement and management. *International Journal of Quality in Health Care* 9 (3): 161-62.

Kimberly, J. R. 1998. La disparition de l'hôpital tel que nous le connaissons. *Gestions Hospitaliéres*, December: 766-9.

Landon, B. E., C. Tobias, and A. M. Epstein. 1998. Quality management by state Medicaid agencies converting to managed care: plans and current practice. *Journal of the American Medical Association* 279: 211-16.

Loughlin, M. 1996. The language of quality. *Journal of Evaluation in Clinical Practice* 2(2):87-95.

McLaughlin, C. P and A. D. Kaluzny. 1997. Total quality management issues in managed care. *Journal of Health Care Finance* 24 (1):10-16.

Mintzberg, H. 1996. Managing government, governing management. *Harvard Business Review*, May —June:75-83.

Mintzberg, H. 1998. Covert leadership: notes on managing professionals. *Harvard Business Review*, November-December:140-47.

Minvielle, E. 1997. Beyond quality management methods: meeting the challenges of health care reform. *International Journal of Quality in Health Care* 9 (3):189-92.

Nonaka, I., and N. Konno. 1998. The concept of "Ba": Building a foundation for knowledge creation. *California Management Review* 40 (3):40-54.

Palmer, R. H. 1997. Using clinical performance measures to drive quality improvement. *Total Quality Management* 8(5): 305-11.

de Pouvourville, G. 1997. Quality of care initiatives in the French context. *International Journal of Quality in Health Care* 9 (3): 163-70.

de Pouvourville, G. 1999. Information systems and quality in health care: A framework for analysis. In *The Quality Imperative*, edited by J. R. Kimberly and E. Minvielle. London: Imperial College Press.

Sales, A., N. Lurie, I. Moscovice, and J. Goes. 1995. Is quality in the eye of the beholder? *Joint Commission Journal on Quality Improvement* 21(5): 219-25.

Shortell, S. M, J. L. O' Brien, J. M. Carman, R. W. Foster, E. F. Hughes, H. Boerslter, and E. J. O' Conner. 1995. Assessing the impact of continuous quality improvement/ total quality management: concept versus implementation. *Health Services Research* 30: 377-401.

Shortell, S. M., R. R. Gillies, and K. J. Devers. 1995. Reinventing the American hospital. *Milbank Quarterly* 73(2):131-60.

Shulkin, D. J. 1997. Quality management in an academic integrated delivery system: The case of the University of Pennsylvania Health System. *International Journal for Quality in Health Care* 9 (3): 171-76.

Shulkin, D. J., and M. S. Joshi. 1999. Quality management at the University of Pennsylvania Health System. In *The Quality Imperative,* edited by J. R. Kimberly and E. Minvielle. London: Imperial College Press.

Silber, J. H., P.R. Rosenbaum, S. V. Williams, R. N. Ross, and J. S. Schwartz. 1997. The relationship between choice of outcome measure and hospital rank in general surgical procedures: Implications for quality assessment. *International Journal for Quality in Health Care* 9(3):193-200.

Sluyter, G. V. 1998. Total quality management in behavioral health care. *New Directions in Mental Health Services* 79: 35-43.

Thomson, R. G. 1998. Quality to the fore in health policy—at last. *British Medical Journal* 17: 95-6.

Thomson, R. G. and A. G. Barton. 1994. Is audit running out of steam? *Quality in Health Care* 3: 225-29.

Thomson, M. A., A. D. Oxman, D. A. Davis, R. B. Haynes, N. Freemantle and E. L. Harvey. 1998a. *Audit and feedback to improve health professional practice and health care outcomes (Part I).* Cochrane Database of Systematic Reviews. Issue 4, 1998.

Thomson, M. A., A. D. Oxman, D. A. Davis, R. B. Haynes, N. Freemantle and E. L. Harvey. 1998b. *Audit and feedback to improve health professional health care outcomes (Part II).* Cochrane Database of Systematic Reviews. Issue 4, 1998.

Tonneau, D. 1997. Management tools and organization as key factors toward quality care: Reflections from experience. *International Journal for Quality in Health Care* 9 (3): 201-5.

Tonneau, D. 1999. Quality management in French hospitals: From implicit concern to radical change. In *The Quality Imperative,* edited by J. R. Kimberly and E. Minvielle. London: Imperial College Press.

Wilson, L. T., and D. Asay. 1999. Putting quality into knowledge management. *Quality Progress*, January: 25-31.

Young, A. P. 1997. Competing ideologies in health care: a personal perspective. *Nursing Ethics* 4(3):191-201.

Young, G. J., M. P. Charns and G. L. Barbour. 1997. Quality improvement in the US Veterans Health Administration. *International Journal for Quality in Health Care* 9 (3): 183-88.

Chapter 10

The Quality Imperative:
Lessons and Potential

Etienne Minvielle and John R. Kimberly

Each of the chapters in this book elaborates, in one way or another, on the quality imperative. The perspectives and experiences presented also raise a number of questions about quality management and the future in healthcare.

In this, the final chapter, our objective is to distill from these different perspectives and experiences, the underlying themes that are associated with the search for quality of care. In so doing, we address the measurement techniques that need to be developed and the actions for improvement that need to be undertaken, as well as the methods of control that need to be designed.

It should be noted that the perspective we adopt is explicitly that of researchers in management and organization theory. Viewing the quality movement through this lens results in new insights: certain assertions are more nuanced and points previously thought secondary are now seen as primordial. For us, the quality movement in healthcare in some respects evokes theories and experiences known for some time in the world of management. In other respects, however, this movement has a highly original "quality", particularly if one goes beyond certain obvious commonalties. We hope, in the following pages, to demonstrate why we believe this to be the case and what the implications may be.

Identifying the underlying themes necessitates, in the first place, establishing benchmarks around the idea of quality of care, for we cannot speak of themes in the absence of widespread and observable practices. The first section of this chapter, therefore, is devoted to terminological and conceptual clarification stimulated by the different definitions proposed by the authors. Understanding such benchmarks allows us to subsequently identify the current challenges that the search for quality must confront. Finally, we argue that far from being a passing fad, the search for quality of care is, from a societal perspective, becoming firmly established, and we suggest certain directions in which the quality movement may move in coming years.

Emerging Trends in the Measurement and Management of Quality

Much has already been said and written about quality of care, its assessment, and its relationships with costs. Do we have anything to add? Precisely because so much has been said, it is useful to return to two basic questions: How, in concrete terms, is quality of care recognized? And, what significant changes can be observed in the quality arena?

Such questions were clearly on the minds of the different chapter authors, as can be seen in the definitions of quality that they propose. They use quite different approaches to framing the concept, a concept that has been frequently criticized for being too broad in scope. Nonetheless, there is agreement among them. They agree—albeit implicitly—that instead of a naive form of pragmatism which would involve a uni-dimensional view of quality, it is preferable to pursue a more nuanced analysis of recent trends. Three such trends can be identified. And in the background, one can see how the approach to analyzing the quality of care has evolved over time from one which is essentially **evaluative**, focusing on professional practices and structures, to one which is more **dynamic** and covers the entire organization of the hospital. Taken together, these three trends suggest an evolution towards a more integrated way of thinking about quality.

Trend 1. Measuring Quality: from Structures to Processes, from Processes to Outcomes

Donabedian's (1988) definition, which distinguishes among the quality of structures, processes and results, constitutes a basic framework for analysis. This return to the "source" is a reminder that recent years have witnessed a subtle transition from an approach based on structures, criticized for its static and bureaucratic character, towards an analysis based on processes and results. Nowadays, assessment of quality is based less and less on criteria such as the number of beds or workforce. It focuses more dynamically on indicators of process and, above all, of results. This transition has been motivated by pressure from accreditation agencies, patients and payers, all of whom, as we noted in Chapter 1, are seeking value.

While this point appears settled, as highlighted by Pouvourville in Chapter 2, the ambiguity between quality as an attribute of the service production process and as an attribute of a result does not appear to be resolved. This is due to the difficulty in establishing links between process and results, when assessing quality. Even in the presence of competent doctors, good management, and optimal organizational structures, the "results" remain largely uncertain, since they are dependent on the behavior of patients. This difficulty distinguishes the health care sector from other sectors. Because of this difficulty, there is a temptation to focus on process, which is simpler to identify and to interpret, rather than on results (Eddy, 1998). Is this argument sufficient to diminish the enthusiasm of certain payers and consumers for the development of indicators of result? Without taking sides in this debate, let us simply note that the construction of intermediate indicators focusing on the results of the process or service, has occasionally led to confusion, as these indicators were inappropriately regarded as measures of results of outcomes.

In parallel, ambiguity persists with regard to the very notion of result. Patient satisfaction, hospital infection rates, and failure rates after major surgery, have all been proposed as measures of results. Gillies and her colleagues make this point in Chapter 5 by distinguishing among four factors that are part of any consideration of the quality of the results of care: health and functional status and quality of life, mortality, morbidity, and quality as perceived by the patient.

These two ambiguities emphasize the extent to which quality remains a multifaceted concept. As the attribute of a process, it is the quality of a service which becomes the subject of analysis; as the result, quality is assessed multidimensionally (Chassin, Galvin and The National Roundtable on Health Care Quality 1998)

Trend 2. Improving Quality: From Professional Practices to Organization

At the same time, organizational factors have been increasingly recognized as influencing the quality of care (Moss, Garside and Dawson 1998). In the context of a system that has become as complex as it is interactive, no single profession alone can claim to be capable of guaranteeing a high level of quality. Patient intakes are becoming faster and faster, involve more and more professionals, and present ever- multiplying courses of action, which are as often diagnostic as they are therapeutic. Faced with such complexity, it is certain that the quality of care provided can no longer be solely the result of the efforts of a single medical specialty, or of the collaboration between a doctor and a nurse in a single department alone. The importance of *organization* in the search for quality of care is not surprising. Experiences in other sectors have demonstrated this [1]. What *may* be surprising, however, is how slowly this fact has become recognized and accepted in the healthcare sector. Two explanations can be offered. One can firstly consider the predominant place of medicine, a place which locates its practices at the heart of quality in the hospital. We should remember here, however, that recognizing the importance of the organization does not mean abandoning all consideration of these practices. It simply involves integrating them into a more general context, that of the organization of work, and moving beyond the boundaries of hospital departments in order to appreciate the overarching importance of serving patients.

An historically weak managerial culture in the healthcare sector also limits the learning from theories and experiences from outside the sector. A widespread belief in the uniqueness of the healthcare sector often leads one to the notion that any transfer of ideas and theories from the business world is impossible. The opposite, however, is also true. The apostles of transfer often display a lack of understanding of the managerial issues that complicate efforts to improve quality in healthcare. QA and CQI procedures are often in conflict since they are based on different principles: the former aiming to develop conformity with pre-established procedures, while the latter calls for the search for continual excellence and development of competencies. From a management perspective, the issue is not the substitution of one for the other, but the understanding of their respective areas of application in hospital activities. QA procedures are perfectly adapted to standardized activities namely, the logistics such as laundry or house-keeping, while CQI is more relevant for the majority of care activities, where one understands the importance of factors which can compromise performance.

Trend 3. From Measurement and Improvement to Improvement and Measurement

The concept of quality refers not only to something that needs to be assessed, but also to a system of action. As something to be assessed, it is now the processes and results more than the structures, which are at the center of analysis (Trend 1). As a system of action, quality is more concerned with improving the organization of productive processes observable at the hospital, such as the prescribing of additional diagnostic tests or prevention of falls (Trend 2). It is then either called QA or CQI and motivates new modes of organization such as cooperative practices, the use of written documents in the context of standardized operating procedures, and new professional practices.

The search for quality thus becomes a cycle comprised of two distinct moments: that of the assessment, and that of the corrective action. In this cycle, the necessity of heightening the concern for evaluation, and the evaluation itself, almost at the same time that the action is conceived and launched, is part of the classic conception (Dumez and Jeunemaître 1998; Chen 1994). One talks of early evaluation or evaluation ex-ante. The history of quality of care shows to what extent, until recently, this conception was favored. In the elaboration of indicators in accordance with the structure-procedure-result pattern or "gold standards" of business practice, the moment of evaluation— quality audit, peer review, accreditation procedures—has most often been preceded by that of action. More than chronological order, it is a relationship of subordination which often establishes itself, with the actions for improving quality needing to be deduced implicitly from the conclusions of the evaluation. Criticisms of procedures for improving quality, of the risks of coercive control linked to compliance with pre-established evaluation criteria (Chassin, Galvin and the National Roundtable on Health Care Quality 1998), and of the orientation towards short term results stemming from use of empirical measures, are evidence of this state of subordination and of its potentially negative consequences.

In response, many newer efforts have highlighted the procedures for improving quality, where the time needed for evaluation influenced the results of such procedures. The change in quality management policy implemented by the University of Pennsylvania is a particularly good illustration of this trend. As reported by David Shulkin and Maulik Joshi in Chapter 7, the first stage was to move from a culture of evaluation and routine response stimulated by external accreditation criteria, to one of internal improvement which the accreditation process helped motivate. In other words, a new mindset replaced the old—improvement of quality replaced conformity to external evaluation criteria as a consequence of the process of accreditation by an outside body. It may be premature to speak of a trend, but we see in this change of mindset at Penn an inversion of the previous relationship of subordination which gave precedence to critical thought over the principle of action. This inversion represents a genuine reorientation of institutional posture toward quality which, should it become more widespread, portends profound change.

Toward a More Integrated Approach

It is interesting to note with Dominique Tonneau in Chapter 3 that, while the theme of quality of care has always been a concern, its status has changed over time, giving rise to different interpretations. The first of these interpretations comes from the medical world. Here, quality equates to good diagnostic and therapeutic practices, founded on scientific methods, and perhaps best expressed through the development of "evidence-based-medicine". Quality has also been used as a rallying cry by nursing bodies in their professional struggle for greater responsibility for patient care. It has also been invoked by administrators concerned with such issues as optimization of structural indicators, compliance with accreditation procedures, or resource allocation criteria within the hospital. Other interpretations, undoubtedly exist as well. But what is important is that all of these interpretations, despite their different emphases, give quality a significant role in internal debates: quality is included in reasoning, whether administrative or professional; and in a very real sense quality becomes an ingredient in political jostling, a sort of totem which is invoked opportunistically in service of diverse special interests.

As a result of these recent developments, summarized in the three trends we discuss, quality seems to have acquired a new status. Professionals naturally tend to associate the search for quality with elaboration of the best diagnostic and therapeutic strategies for care, thereby demonstrating the importance of the organizational context in which such strategies must be implemented (Trend 2). Alternatively, faced with a reading that focuses on the optimization of structural indicators and the importance of the evaluative phase, emphasis is placed on the internal management of the activities of patient care, evaluated by results (Trends 1 and 3).

These trends suggest a new approach to the quality of care. It becomes a vehicle for rationalizing hospital activity; the search for it leads to the development of new modes of work organization, and to improved care of patients and understanding of their link with changes in results. In this approach, it is no longer a case of opposition between professional and administrative staffs, medical decisions and organizational context, or time of evaluation and of action, but of integration of these different components into a single framework, thereby encouraging a more holistic perspective. In our view, these changes will, in the long run, lead to a more integrated approach to quality.

This will not happen quickly or easily. The organizational logic on which this new approach relies, remains to a large extent incomplete. There is also no guarantee that the changes brought about by this evolution will be accepted. The chapter by Gillies and her colleagues shows clearly that behind this process are groups of actors with distinct interests. Furthermore, the indicators that are supposed to allow regular evaluation in themselves raise methodological issues. Finally, beyond the rhetoric is the question of the real benefit for the patient.

The Challenges

What, then, are the challenges that this approach to the quality of care must confront as it becomes more fully elaborated? Although the need to develop procedures for improving and evaluating quality is widely recognized, failures in their implementation have also been perceived for some time, as Len Lerer points out in the previous chapter and as Loizeau (1996) has noted elsewhere. Poor credibility and few permanent effects on the hospital's day-to-day operation quality are but two examples of the kind of flawed implementation that has created a residue of disenchantment with initiatives and a sense that these initiatives consist only of a series of tools bereft of any overarching strategic or philosophical cohesion. The "seven perversions" in the application of quality approaches in healthcare described by Tabet and Téboul (1998) are eloquent testimony to the magnitude of the challenge of "getting it right".

Simply lamenting these "perversions", however, is not enough. They tend to be present whenever managerial innovation is introduced (Kimberly, 1981; Abrahamson, 1991). On the other hand, the issue cannot be reduced simply to the study of "techniques" that have already been introduced elsewhere; it really is located more generally at the level of organizational learning in the context of the introduction of new practices. From this perspective, the search for quality presents, apart from any effects of ideas in vogue, the foundations for a new management philosophy, as Dominique Tonneau suggests in Chapter 3. This new philosophy includes new forms of medical-administrative exchanges, new approaches to looking after patients and even new forms of control. Understandably, this new philosophy begets numerous challenges at the organizational, managerial, methodological and economic levels. Although each may require specific responses, they are also systematically connected.

They are all parts of the same puzzle and, as we noted in Chapter 1, fit together along two axes. One axis is organizational and concerns processes. Improving quality depends both on the definition of a context for organizational analysis and practices of change management. The other axis is technical, and considers quality as an object to be controlled through use of reliable measurements.

Elaborating an Organizational Framework

Transversality, dysfunctions, and cooperation are all terms which have become part of the quality lexicon, and they have one thing in common. They all place the internal organization of hospitals at the center of analysis—improved quality is achieved through organizational change.

A number of improvements have been made under this banner—better reception of patients, reorganization of the O.R., or improved dispensing of medicines—and their importance should not be under-estimated. The hospital is nourished by these micro-innovations developed in daily work. But true quality management is more than this. The organization of work provides a framework for analysis which includes all these improvements, but which also includes more general considerations such as the system's rigidity and partitioning, the central position given to patients and their treatment, and the flows of information within the system. It is the integration of **all** these elements within a single framework that gives the focus on organization its added value. From this point of view, several benchmarks can be provided, with the help of theories and concepts from the management sciences.

To begin, we evoke a fundamental principle of management: an organizational response only has meaning in reference to an activity. Introducing more standardization or more autonomy does not have meaning in any absolute sense, but only in relation to the characteristics of an activity, understood as a productive process. In this respect, taking care of patients can be characterized as a process where, as Len Lerer argues in the previous chapter, the uniqueness of cases remains a basic datum. In order to symbolize this uniqueness, Corbin and Strauss (1988) speak of the patient trajectory. At the same time, these trajectories cannot be managed on a "craft" basis. Many patients are hospitalized simultaneously. Their length of stay also tends to be increasingly brief. The challenge confronting the modern hospital can best be described as that of mass customization, of managing uniqueness on a large scale (Minvielle, 1996).

This problem is not limited to hospitals and patient care. Many recent experiences in service industries and in manufacturing highlight the need to take aspects such as variety and responsiveness into account when developing production processes[2]. Even if the determinants are different, studying the responses which were proposed is instructive. These disclose the "rise to power" of the notion of flexibility, *"a concept which is progressively becoming one of the major objectives of organizations in their experiments with higher levels of complexity"* (Cohendet and Llerena, 1999). The notion of flexibility must be understood here at organizational level. Applying the principle of flexible organization in the context of the hospital implies two major orientations:

First of all, the search for flexibility does not, perforce, contradict the need to maintain a certain degree of standardization. There is a tendency to invoke the Taylorist character of hospital organization when seeking to justify the need for greater flexibility in the work of professionals. This tendency both misinterprets the foundation of scientific management[3], and secondly, introduces opposition precisely where the objective is to seek complementarity. Martin Charns and his colleagues, for example, show clearly in Chapter 4 how the challenge of coordination is not to oppose "standardized procedures and control" versus "informal interactions and autonomy", but to know how to accommodate these two approaches in the same framework. The objective of flexible organization is therefore to find a balance between the development of standardization and programming on one hand,

and the development of autonomy and more informal practices on the other.

Second, this search for "flexibility" is played out in the context of an organization, which depends above all on the people within it. In other words, the organization only reasons in terms of the human capital represented by all the professionals participating on a daily basis in the activity of patient care. This fact has the effect of placing the concepts of know-how and organizational learning at the core of the flexible organization (Nonaka 1994; Argyris and Schön 1980). As highlighted by Hatchuel and Weil (1992): "if the reduction of uncertainty or diversity is necessary, when they are there, there are not many alternatives to a sharing of know-how which enables each actor, not only to do what is asked of him, but also to be ready to respond to what has not been anticipated, and even better, to understand the consequences of this unforeseen event for his colleagues".

Several types of organizational know-how can thus be envisaged: the know-how associated with mastery of a task: the know-how associated with effective coordination of activities, the know-how associated with an effective response to unanticipated occurrences, the know-how associated with effective identification of organizational problems, and finally, the know-how associated with effective empathy, which can be used by nursing staff in order to teach a patient how to be an actor in his own "trajectory". It is through their collective motivation that nursing professionals are able to engage effectively in an activity, part of which lies outside any formal measures or explicit rules.

Organizational Change: New Practices of Management

The definition of a new organizational framework is only a first step. For it to be adopted, it is necessary to anticipate, as it is being elaborated, the appropriate conditions for change. The organizational changes required by adoption of this framework challenge existing management practices in the hospital, as can be seen from the experiences and research reported in the various chapters of this book.

Gillies and her colleagues propose a way to rank such management practices. This approach emphasizes the need to assess the alignment among several dimensions—structural, strategic, technical and cultural—in order to analyze the implementation of CQI. David Shulkin and Maulik Joshi highlight different key factors for success in the experience of the University of Pennsylvania—the role of leadership, the importance of structural organization, methods of measurement, and the manner of reporting on actions undertaken internally. Isabelle Durand-Zaleski and Pierre Durieux in their chapter, and Gérard de Pouvourville in his, point out the central importance of the development of information systems. Durand-Zaleski and Durieux emphasize the necessity for autonomy in the management of such information systems in relation to the administration which is often in charge of them, while de Pouvourville questions the advantages of investing in new information systems, when existing medico-administrative databases provide the platform for substantial analyses. The factors noted above, do not constitute an exhaustive list, although they do help, in conjunction with others, to locate hospitals' posture toward quality between two extremes; the status quo and profound change. In the former, the structures involved with quality are established before projects and power plays are introduced to the detriment of transversal reasoning, the operation of information systems in the search for quality remains under administrative control, and pursuit of a good accreditation score becomes an end in itself rather than a tool for internal self-evaluation.

In the latter, the reasoning on the structures to be implemented is then the subject of decentralized coordination in line with a pre-established policy. The forms of power are placed at the service of the procedure —all players share responsibility for quality; measures are subject to feedback sessions; information systems are managed in a quality promoting manner; budgets permit variation; professional structures have flexibility and quality becomes an incentive.

In this approach, the involvement of the medical and nursing corps in policies of improving quality is essential. The importance of this involvement is well-illustrated by the experiences reported from the American (Chapters 4 and 7) as well as French (Chapter 6) points of view. The underlying argument is part of the conventional wisdom. This involvement is necessary since doctors and nursing staff remain the real "operators" of quality. And it is in the day-to-day practices, on the floors of the care units themselves, that the success or failure of these procedures is played out. Experience shows the pay-offs from investment in policies of quality improvement (such as the compulsory quality training program for faculty physicians at the University of Pennsylvania) which enhance this involvement. Surprisingly, until recently the role of professionals in the production of quality was under-emphasized, if not ignored. As noted earlier, organizational effectiveness depends above all on the level of the women and men involved in it. Could it be that the quality imperative has led to the rediscovery of the importance of human capital?

Control by Quality

Alan Meynard (1998), in retracing the history of the British NHS and U.S.-style managed care, emphasizes how much more evident control by quality is in rhetoric than in practice. This observation is probably true for most industrialized countries.

The author's explanation is that the search for quality tends to be overshadowed by policies for controlling public spending. In other words, cuts in public spending are made at the expense of commitment to a high level of quality. For this to change, the author argues that the trade-off between quality and cost needs to be clarified, and the idea that the improvement of quality inevitably involves higher costs needs to be debunked. In some cases, improving quality and reducing costs can go hand in hand, particularly when managing costs due to the overuse of services. Additional investments do, however, appear necessary in order to reduce misuses, and above all to deal with under-use (Bodenheimer, 1999).

From an economic point of view, Chilingerian in Chapter 8 and de Pouvourville in Chapter 2 mention the ambiguity where the control of costs, the search for efficiency, and the search for quality may be contradictory. When seen as a result, quality appears to be linked to allocative efficiency: if one knows how to measure it, this constitutes a criterion of performance in the allocation of resources between producers. When seen as an attribute of the process, quality is linked to the notion of technical efficiency, understood as the best possible combination of available resources. De Pouvourville argues that in this case, the cost-quality trade-off reverts to that of a conventional production process with four possible combinations. In his chapter, Chilingerian shows how DEA methods can relate technical efficiency to quality in terms of result. By defining a production function which links a combination of resources at the level of results, it becomes possible to analyze the relationship between quality and efficiency.

These experiences and the perspectives on which they are based are clearly exceptional. Their broader diffusion depends on the encouragement of contractual practices among payers, providers, patients and public authorities, practices common in the majority of developed countries, to fill in the gap between a focus on efficiency and the search for quality.

Measures of Quality and Performance: From a Piecemeal to a Multidimensional Approach

Issues relating to the control of quality shape the methodological questions. The measurement of quality necessary for control can be envisaged alone, or in relation with costs, and more generally with different attributes of hospital performance. At each of these stages, the search for quality finds itself confronted with metrological difficulties. Finally, it is important to add that, whatever the level of analysis, there are also problems with the methods which may be used to obtain the information.

The metrological issues specific to the measurement of quality, although not resolved, are certainly well-known. Outcomes measurement has become a field of research in itself. In Chapter 8, Chilingerian points out a number of current weaknesses

First, there is no overarching interpretative framework which enables an observed level of result to be linked to a level of performance: certain Quality Outcome Ratios are high and others not, but there are no means of verifying whether better results could be obtained, or whether the observed difference is justified;

Second, the ratios between observed and expected values generally reflect average trends, but do not indicate best practice;

And finally, the multiplicity of ratios resulting from taking into account the multidimensional character of quality makes practical application difficult.

DEA type methods make it possible to address these issues by defining a production function. They are thus likely to be used more extensively in the future since they can easily be applied to the healthcare sector where complex "technologies" require that the constraints of the econometric model be relaxed.

The notion of a trade-off between cost and quality poses another methodological challenge, that of organizational performance and its measurement. The conventional view of performance in organizational theory relies on three principles: (1) organizations pursue multiple and often contradictory objectives (Cameron 1986); (2) the "results" from some types of organizations are more easily quantifiable than those from others; and (3) every organization has multiple stakeholders, each of which judges the organization's performance in accordance with its own priorities and in terms of its own perceptions. There are therefore several criteria for evaluating organizational performance (Cameron 1986, Quinn and Rohrbaugh 1983). The multidimensional character of organizational performance in general helps to explain the existence of several definitions of performance in the specific case of hospitals. Further complicating the issue are generic difficulties in measuring results in hospitals to begin with, poor definition of objectives, and the particular importance of interest groups (Sicotte et al. 1998).

It is no doubt illusory to believe that all relevant dimensions of hospital performance could be incorporated in a single framework. On the other hand, there is a fundamental need to develop the concept further by going beyond the relationship between costs and quality, and taking into account other aspects described as fundamental in the analysis of organizational performance, such as the hospital's adaptation to its surroundings (Pfeffer and Salancik 1978), and its capacity to respond to the interests of various influential groups of actors (Scott, 1981). This development would have the virtue of making the trade-offs between quality and other criteria more explicit.

Whatever the methodological difficulties involved in the measurement of quality and performance, there is still the challenge of how best to use the results obtained. Among the many approaches being tried, the example described by Shulkin and Joshi in Chapter 7 appears particularly promising. They highlight the potential of using scorecards, which by definition include many different indicators of performance. Use of scorecards as method of presentation helps to avoid preoccupation with a single criterion and to facilitate the differential weighting of multiple objectives. The benchmarking approach used, whether internal or external to the hospital, also shows the importance of feed-back when results are incorporated into a comparative analysis. It becomes a motivator for the improvement of quality, and for the improvement of performance more generally. And, in the light of the discussion in Chapter

5 by Charns and his colleagues, it also constitutes an excellent method for identifying the most effective forms of organization.

Going beyond the specific techniques used, there is also the question of level of restitution: from the "micro" of the population of a hospital department to the "macro" of the determining factors for the health of a population on a national scale, not forgetting the "meso" of hospital and accreditation agency analyses. Here again we see the need for clarification of the levels of analysis, their respective use, and their coherence.

Future Directions

The measurement and management of quality constitutes a significant challenge for hospitals, a challenge which will be attenuated in the future by many factors: by discoveries, for example, in molecular biology which will transform today's medical knowledge; by the affirmation of evidence-based-medicine; and, unfortunately, by the appearance of new risks as yet unknown. Only in the future will we know what balance is ultimately struck in the search for quality among professional, administrative and organizational interests. And only then will we see how CQI and TQM approaches have fared. Will they have taken hold and become part of a new management philosophy or will they prove to have been a passing fad, in the end having had little impact on conventional approaches to producing quality? Only time will tell.

But no matter how this evolves, we would like to conclude by drawing the reader's attention to two issues which, although perhaps not at the center of debate today, will be in the very near future. These are the development of a broader perspective on quality, and the patient's potential role in this movement.

From a Hospital to a Societal Perspective

A common feature of current thinking about quality is the central importance of the organization of work. Quality is no longer seen as simply a matter of professional expertise or of compliance with administrative rules. It is seen as an objective for the rationalization of the hospital's production system. Certain of the experiences reported in this book exemplify this broadened perspective, a perspective which is moving in three directions:

First there is an increasing awareness of the need to go beyond the hospital's boundaries and to think about care on a broader basis. The notion of a care network illustrates this trend. As mentioned by Tonneau in Chapter 3, this is not a new idea. Emergency and ambulance services, for example, have tried to combine their efforts to create more coordinated care networks for some time. This theme has long been the subject of experiments and today the notion of network has become central to thinking about health policy and planning. This means that the organizational lessons likely to be learned through efforts to measure and manage quality do not stop at the hospital's doors. The patient's trajectory continues after hospitalization, and this obvious reality must be incorporated in thinking about quality. In brief, the search for quality affects the widest area of care being offered (Kimberly 1998). What influence will this broader perspective have on the methods of organizing trajectories, or on the definition of performance indicators? If the framing of the problem does not change, it is difficult to anticipate the impact of organizations in which the links among professionals will inevitably be more numerous but also looser, in terms of length of relationships, loyalty or processing of information. Let us simply emphasize that quality will depend even more on mechanisms of cooperation among these professionals, and thus a willingness to accept and use them.

Second, in their chapter, Shulkin and Joshi use recent developments in the policy for improving quality at the University of Pennsylvania to show another aspect of quality: a policy geared initially toward improvement of patient care has evolved in the direction of a policy for improvement of a population's level of health (Shortell et al. 1995). This evolution presupposes the integration of primary care, follow-up care and long stays, and no longer focuses solely on emergency care.

Third, we see a transition from concern with quality of care to concern for quality of health. Even if it is widely recognized today that an individual's state of health does not depend solely on the quality of care provided to him, the conditions for the transition from the search for quality of care to quality of health remain largely unknown. Many factors including personal attributes such as social status, lifestyles and living conditions, are sources of variation in the state of health, and are independent of care. What changes will be necessary to improve a population's health, that is, to limit "the wear and tear caused by various aspects of living conditions"? There is no way of telling at present, but responding to such questions in the future is, as Contandriopoulos (1999) argues, "*the* challenge for public health".

These three directions together define the contours of a new perspective to which quality may be applied in the near future. From a largely hospital perspective, focusing on remedial care, considerations of quality are likely to move toward a broader societal perspective integrating aspects of prevention and focusing on health rather than exclusively on illness.

Driven by the Consumer: Rhetoric and Reality

We have saved you and us—the consumers of healthcare and the arbiters of health on an individual basis—for last to highlight the complex linkage between the individual and the search for quality. The place that we have in the movement is paradoxical, since it is both central and virtual.

It is **central**, first of all, in considering you and us as users "benefiting" from the policies for improving quality. This theme has become a *leitmotiv* adopted by the public authorities as well as by many hospital management teams. Surveys to measure satisfaction and complaints have multiplied. Efforts to "humanize" the process have also been made at the different stages of the patient trajectory. Legal and statutory regulations protecting the patients' rights have been strengthened, particularly the obligation to inform the patient. And even if there may be some gaps between theory and practice, the result is that the quality imperative has fostered a strong institutional dynamic promoting the patient's comfort and safety.

It is **virtual** as well, in terms of real participation in the search for quality. Many analyses of quality remain quantitative and say little about the interaction, at an individual level, between the patient and the service system (Galvin 1998). As Lerer puts it in the previous chapter: "The failure to recognize that the business of health care is the improvement of health status at an individual level inevitably leads to conditions under which quality initiatives cannot succeed". Similarly, many analyses have nothing to say about the level of quality "desired" by consumers, heard not only as consumers of services, but also as citizens attentive to the quality of health services. It is therefore both as a customer and as a citizen that our voice needs to be heard in the search for quality.

For many reasons, current discussions about the "new health consumer" are largely rhetorical. However, we are optimistic that, overtime, the rhetoric will become reality. In our view, the current panoply of initiatives around the new health consumer signal a trend, not a fad, and this trend will only further reinforce the quality imperative.

Notes

[1] Deming (1986), for example, estimates that 85% of malfunctions observed in businesses are organizational in origin against only 15% involving professional failures.

[2] As an illustration, if we recall that in 1908 Ford offered the Model T in a single option, nowadays Peugeot offers more than 10,000 combinations of its 306 model.

[3] Maybe because there has never been a system of autonomous organizational reasoning in hospitals, as could be envisaged in the research departments designed by Taylor. As a general rule, a poor understanding of the organizational and social impact of Taylor's work has often resulted in any form of standardization being assimilated to it in an exaggerated manner, where the issue is at the level of design, in a scientific predetermination of the work (see de Montmollin 1981).

References

Abrahamson, E. 1991. Managerial fads and fashions: The diffusion and rejection of innovations. *Academy of Management Review* 16:586-612.

Argyris, C., and D. Schön. 1978. *Organizational learning: a theory of action perspective*. New York:Addison-Wesley.

Bodenheimer, T. 1999. The American health care system. The movement for improved quality in health care. *New England Journal of Medicine* 340: 488-92.

Cameron, K. 1986. A study of organizational effectiveness and its predictors. *Management Science* 32(1):87-112.

Chassin, M. R. 1998. Is health care ready for Six Sigma quality? *Milbank Quarterly* 76 (4):565-91.

Chassin, M. R., R. W. Galvin and The National Roundtable on Health Care Quality. 1998. The urgent need to improve health care quality: Institute of Medicine Roundtable on Health Care Quality. *Journal of the American Medical Association* 280:1000-5.

Chen, H. T. 1994. Theory-driven Evaluations: Need, difficulties and options. *Evaluation Practice* 15(1):79-82.

Cohendet, P., and P. Llerena. 1999. Flexibilité et modes d'organisation. *Revue Française de Gestion* 123:72-80.

Contandriopoulos. A. P.1999. Pourquoi est-il si difficile de faire ce qui est souhaitable? Quelques idées sur la transformation des systèmes de santé. Conférence "Le managed care et les NOPS", Département de la santé et de l'action sociale du canton de Vaud, Lausanne.

Corbin, J. and A. Strauss. 1988. *Unending Work and Care*. San Francisco: Jossey-Bass Publishers.

Deming, W. E. 1986. *Out of Crisis*. Massachusetts: Cambridge University Press.

Donabedian, A. 1988. The quality of care: how can it be assessed? *Journal of the American Medical Association* 260:1743-48.

Dumez, H., and A. Jeunemâitre 1998. *Évaluer l'action publique*. Paris: Logiques Politiques, L'Harmattan.

Eddy, D. M. 1998. Performance measurement: Problems and solutions. *Health Affairs* 17(4):7-25.

Galvin, R.S. 1997. Are performance measures relevant? *Health Affairs* 17(4): 29-31.

Hatchuel, A. and L. B.Weil. 1992. *L'expert et le système*. Paris: Economica.

Kimberly, J.R. 1981. Managerial innovation. In P.C. Nystrom and W.H. Starbuck (Eds.) *Handbook of Organizational Design*. Oxford, Oxford University Press: 84-104.

Kimberly, J. R. 1998. La disparition de l'hôpital tel que nous le connaissons. *Gestions Hospitaliéres*, December:766-9.

Loizeau, D. 1996. L'effondrement tranquille de la gestion de la qualité: résultats d'une étude réalisée dans douze hôpitaux publics au Québec. *Ruptures* 3:187-208.

Minvielle, E. 1996. Gérer la singularité à grande échelle. *Revue Française de Gestion* 109:119-24

Meynard, A. 1998. Competition and quality: Rhetoric and reality. *International Journal for Quality in Health Care* 10(5):379-83.

Moss, F., P. Garside, and S. Dawson. 1998. Organizational change: the key to quality improvement. *Quality in Health Care* Suppl: S1-S2.

de Montmollin, M. 1981. *Le Taylorisme à visage humain*. Paris:Presses Universitaires de France.

Nonaka, I. 1994. A dynamic theory of organizational knowledge creation. *Organization Science* 5(1):102-13

Pfeffer, J., and G. R. Salancik. 1978. *The external control of organizations*. New York: Harper and Row

Quinn, R. E. and J. Rohrbaugh. 1983. A spatial model of effectiveness criteria: Towards a competing values approach to organizational analysis. *Management Science* 29(3):363-77.

Scott, W. R. 1981. Organization: Rational, natural, and open systems. Englewood Cliffs, N.J.: Prentice-Hall.2d Ed, 1987.

Shortell, S. M, J. L. O' Brien, J. M. Carman, R. W. Foster, E. F. Hughes, H. Boerslter, and E. J. O' Conner. 1995. Assessing the impact of continuous quality improvement/total quality management: concept versus implementation. *Health Services Research* 30: 377-401.

Sicotte, C., F. Champagne, A. P. Contandripoulos, et al. 1998. A conceptual framework for the analysis of health care. *Management Research* 11: 24-48.

Tabet, J. and J. Teboul. 1998. *The seven perversions of quality*. INSEAD Working Paper, Fontainebleau, France: INSEAD.

Notes on Contributors

Peter P. Budetti is the Director of the Institute for Health Services Research and Policy Studies at Northwestern University, Chicago and Evanston. He is a Professor with joint tenure in the Department of Preventive Medicine and in the Kellogg Graduate School of Management, and holds an appointment as Professor in the School of Law.

Martin Charns is Director of the Management Decision and Research Center, a research, consulting, technology assessment, and information dissemination organization in the Health Services Research and Development Service of the Department of Veterans Affairs, created to bridge the gap between research and practice. He is also Professor and Director, Program on Health Policy and Management at the Boston University School of Public Health. His research interests focus on organization design and change.

Jon A. Chilingerian is Associate Professor of Management, Director of the MBA Program and Co-Director of the Doctoral Program in Health Services Research at Brandeis University. He is a visiting professor of health care management and organizational behavior at INSEAD (1998-2000). He received his Ph.D. in Management from MIT's Sloan School of Management and teaches graduate courses and executive education sessions in Organizational Theory and Managerial Behavior and Management of Health Care Organizations.

Jennifer Daley is a member of the Department of Medicine and the Health Services Research and Development Service, Boston Healthcare System, Department of Veterans Affairs. She is also Associate Professor of Medicine, Harvard Medical School, and Director, Center for Health System Design and Evaluation, Institute for Health Policy, Massachusetts General Hospital/Partners Healthcare System. Her research interests include access to healthcare services, assessments of patient satisfaction and patient-reported quality of care, quality measurement and management of surgical patients, and the impact of cost reduction and improved efficiency on the quality of health care.

David Dranove is the Richard Paget Distinguished Professor of Management and Strategy and chair of the Department of Management and Strategy at Northwestern University's Kellogg Graduate School of Management. He is also Professor of Health Services Management. He has a Ph.D. in Business Economics from Stanford University. Professor Dranove's research and teaching focus on problems in industrial organization and business strategy with an emphasis on the health care industry.

Isabelle Durand-Zaleski is Professor at the University of Paris XII and Chief of the Evaluation Department of the Henri Mondor hospital, Paris. She has a Masters degree in Public Policy from the Institut d'Etudes Politiques de Paris, a Masters degree in Public Health, Health Policy and Management from Harvard University and a PhD in Economics from the University of Paris IX. Her current research interests include the economic evaluation of health care, accreditation and the development of practice guidelines.

Pierre Durieux is responsible of the clinical evaluation and quality assurance program of Cochin Hospital, one of the major Assistance Publique-Hôpitaux de Paris (AP-HP) hospitals. He is associate Professor of Public Health at University Pierre et Marie Curie (Paris VI). He has a Masters degree in Public Health from the Johns Hopkins School of Hygiene and Public Health. Dr Durieux was previously based at ANDEM (French National Agency for the Development of Medical Evaluation). He has participated in several EC and WHO groups in Technology Assessment and clinical guideline development.

Robin R. Gillies is a Research Specialist at the University of California, Berkeley, and the Project Director of the Center for Organized Delivery Systems and the Physician-System Alignment Study. She is co-author of *Remaking Health Care in America*. Along with her colleagues, she has received article of the year awards from both the American College of Healthcare Executives and the National Institute for Health Care Management.

William G. Henderson is Director of the Hines Cooperative Studies Program Coordinating Center, Research Professor at the Institute for Health Care Policy and Research, Northwestern University, and Adjunct Associate Professor in the Biometry and Epidemiology Program, School of Public Health, University of Illinois.

Cheng-Fang Huang is a Statistical Analyst/Programmer in the Department of Preventive Medicine at Northwestern University. She has worked as a consultant statistician on several medical and public health research projects. She is a co-author of several papers with medical investigators.

Edward F. X. Hughes is the founder and immediate past director of a University-based policy research center as well as Professor of Health Services Management and Management and Strategy at the Kellogg Graduate School of Management, Northwestern University. Hughes is a frequent author and speaker on managed care and national health policy issues, and a convener and facilitator of managed care meetings.

Maulik S. Joshi is the Senior Director of Quality for the University of Pennsylvania (Penn) Health System and a Senior Fellow at the Leonard Davis Institute of Health Economics. Mr. Joshi leads the quality management program for the Penn Health System, including quality improvement and outcomes management. Mr. Joshi serves on committees with the Institute for Healthcare Improvement, the Agency for Health Care Policy and Research, and the National Committee for Quality Assurance.

Shukri F. Khuri is Chief of the Department of Surgery, Boston Healthcare System, the Department of Veterans Affairs, Professor of Surgery, Harvard Medical School, and Associate Chief of Surgery, Brigham and Women's Hospital. Dr. Khuri's interests include basic research on cardiac function, clinical science research on myocardial protection, revascularization and prevention of arrhythmogenesis, and health services research on outcomes in patients undergoing surgery.

John R. Kimberly is Henry Bower Professor in the Departments of Management and Health Care Systems in the Wharton School and Professor of Sociology in the School of Arts and Sciences at the University of Pennsylvania. He is also Visiting Professor of Organizational Behaviour and Novartis Professor in Healthcare Management at INSEAD in Fontainebleau, France. He is interested in problems of innovation and change in healthcare, in the dimensions and dynamics of organizational identity in organizations in general, and in how individuals are responding to the "new employment relationship".

Leonard B. Lerer is Research Fellow at the INSEAD Healthcare Management Initiative. He is a physician with post-graduate training in epidemiology, biostatistics and forensic pathology. He has an MBA from the University of Cape Town. Dr Lerer is a member of expert panels convened by the World Bank and World Health Organization. His main research interest is in the application of strategic management theory in the public and private health sectors.

Etienne Minvielle is a researcher at the Centre National de la Recherche Scientifique (C.N.R.S) in Paris. He received his medical degree in Public Health from the Medical School of Paris. He is a graduate of the Ecole Supérieure Sciences Economiques et Commerciales (E.S.S.E.C) and obtained his PhD in Management from Ecole Polytechnique. His research concentrates on new organizational design for managing the process of care, health service users and the measurement of hospital performance. He is currently a Fellow at the Centre de Recherche en Economie de la Santé (INSERM-CNRS), and has appointments with the Assistance Publique-Hôpitaux de Paris and Ecole Nationale de la Santé Publique.

Gérard de Pouvourville is Research Director at the French National Centre for Scientific research. He is currently the Director of Group IMAGE, the health services research group of the National School of Public Health. He sits on the Health Information System National Advisory Council. He has conducted research on hospital management and information systems, and on the diffusion of innovation in the health care industry. He has also been an advisor to the French Ministry of Health for the conception and implementation of a case mix adjusted prospective budgeting system.

Alfred W. Rademaker is a biostatistician and a Professor in the Department of Preventive Medicine, Northwestern University Medical School. He is also a senior biostatistician in The Robert H. Lurie Comprehensive Cancer Center of Northwestern University. He is actively involved in cancer clinical trials as well as studies of head and neck cancer, Alzheimer's disease, chronic fatigue syndrome and health services. His interests are focussed on clinical trial and survey study design, sample size determination and statistical analysis of multivariate data.

Katherine S. E. Reynolds was the Project Coordinator for the National Study for the Assessment of the Impact and Implementation of Continuous Quality Improvement. Currently she working at the Institute for Health Services Research and Policy Studies at Northwestern University developing systems to improve and enhance the quality of data collection and tracking for several outcomes studies. She gained her nursing qualifications in London and has a variety of acute care experience with a critical care focus. She continues to practice in the acute care setting.

Stephen M. Shortell is the Blue Cross of California Distinguished Professor of Health Policy and Management and Professor of Organization Behavior at the School of Public Health, University of California, Berkeley. He has been the recipient of many awards including the distinguished Baxter Prize for his contributions to health services research, the Gold Medal Award from the American College of Healthcare, and the Distinguished Investigator Award from the Association for Health Services Research. He is the editor of Health Services Research and is an elected member of the Institute of Medicine of the National Academy of Sciences.

David J. Shulkin is the Chief Medical Officer and Chief Quality Officer of the University of Pennsylvania Health System. Dr. Shulkin leads Penn's efforts in building an integrated delivery system through developing and managing disease management, quality systems, managed care operations, and medical management capabilities. Dr. Shulkin is a Senior Fellow at the Leonard Davis Institute for Health Economics, a Fellow at the Center for Biostatistics and Clinical Epidemiology, and the Institute on Aging at Penn. Dr. Shulkin is a board certified internist and an Associate Professor of Medicine.

Dominique Tonneau is Professor at the Ecole des Mines de Paris and a researcher at the Centre de Gestion Scientifique. His research aims to develop procedures, information systems and strategic tools to assist managers in daily operations. He has led studies dealing with management issues and quality policy in industry and public organizations, with a particular focus on hospitals.

He is a member of various committees in the French Ministry of Health and an adviser to major French hospitals on physician management training.

Gary Young is senior researcher at the Management Decision and Research Center, Health Services Research and Development Service, Department of Veteran's Affairs. He is also associate professor of health services and co-director of the Program on Health Policy and Management at the Boston University School of Public health. His research focuses on organizational, managerial, and legal issues associated with the delivery of healthcare services.

Index